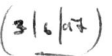

MRCP Part I Paediatric MCQ Revision Book

Ian Maconochie MB BS MRCP(Ire)
*Honorary Registrar,
Department of Paediatrics,
St Mary's Hospital, London.*

Jo Wilmshurst MB BS MRCP
*Paediatric Registrar
The Childrens' Hospital Lewisham,
London.*

© 1995 PASTEST
Knutsford
Cheshire
Telephone: 01565 755226

All rights reserved. No part of this publication may be reproduced, stored in a retrieval system, or transmitted, in any form or by any means, electronic, mechanical, photocopying, recording or otherwise, without the prior permission of the copyright owner.

First edition 1995

Reprinted 1995

ISBN 0 906896 39 8

A catalogue record for this book is available from the British Library.

Typeset by Carnegie Publishing, 18 Maynard Street, Preston.
Printed and bound by Hobbs The Printers, Totton, Hants.

CONTENTS

Correct answers and teaching notes follow the questions in each chapter.

Introduction	iv
MCQ Technique	v
Reading and Reference Books	vii
Anatomy	1
Physiology	6
Biochemistry	19
Pharmacology	23
Embryology	29
Immunology	33
Nutrition	37
Ear, Nose and Throat	41
Neonatology	45
Respiratory Disease	54
Haematology	62
Oncology	69
Cardiology	75
Renal Disease	82
Gastroenterology	90
Metabolic Disorders	99
Endocrinology	105
Neurology	114
Childhood Development	126
Ophthalmology	130
Rheumatology/Orthopaedics	134
Infectious Diseases	143
Dermatology	153
Genetics and Syndromes	159
Statistics and Epidemiology	165
Immunisation	171
Surgery	177
Psychiatry/Psychosocial Paediatrics	181
Accident and Emergency	188
Practice Exam	192
Appendix: Revision Lists	224
Revision Index	225

INTRODUCTION

Membership of the Royal College of Physicians is a prerequisite to higher training in paediatrics and requires the successful completion of Part 1 and Part 2 of the Paediatric 'Membership' exams.

The MCQs used in this new book have been specially written to provide the best possible revision guide for MRCP Part 1 Paediatric candidates. The authors have focused on "favourite" topics based on careful study of the Royal College Paediatric examination papers which have appeared since the new examination was introduced in October 1993. The questions are arranged by subject enabling candidates to use this book as part of a structured revision plan. Basic sciences are emphasised with chapters on anatomy, physiology, biochemistry and pharmacology included.

Correct answers and expanded teaching notes are included for every question. The authors have included many "lists" which candidates will find invaluable for fast effective revision. An index for speedy reference to these lists is provided in the appendix on page 224.

This book culminates with a complete Practice Exam of 60 paediatric questions which is designed to be completed under timed conditions. It is important to note that the official exam consists of 30 paediatric and 30 general medicine questions but for revision purposes we are providing a full practice exam of paediatric questions exclusively. This combination of chapters concentrating on specific subject areas followed by the opportunity to practice MCQ exam technique will enable candidates to isolate and eliminate any weak areas of knowledge before the examination day.

The authors have deliberately included questions which candidates may find demanding. The book has been read by a number of recent exam candidates who have agreed that this is a stimulating and helpful policy which ensures that candidates prepare thoroughly for this important exam.

Good luck when you take the examination.

Acknowledgements

The authors wish to thank Dr Nigel Klein for his invaluable assistance in this project. We would also like to thank the MRCP 1 Paediatric candidates who read this book during its production for their kind words and constructive comments.

MCQ TECHNIQUE

The MRCP Part 1 Paediatric exam is highly competitive. There is no fixed pass mark, instead there is a fixed pass *rate* of 35%. This means that 65% of candidates must fail the examination. To pass the exam you must outshine your colleagues. PasTest revision books and courses are designed to give ambitious candidates a competitive edge.

How To Use This Book
This book contains over 300 MCQs arranged by subject followed by one complete Practice Exam. By working systematically through the book chapter by chapter you will be able to pinpoint areas which you find most demanding. Reasons for getting an answer wrong include poor knowledge, memory at fault, misunderstood the question, hasty/wild guess. It is important for you to understand *why* you got a question wrong so that you can learn from your mistakes. By marking clearly all the questions that you got wrong or declined to answer you can then refresh your memory with the explanations given here or read up on the specific topic in depth using a textbook. Structured revision of this kind enables candidates to focus on individual subject areas and to become familiar with "favourite" Royal College questions and topics.

You should set aside 2½ hours to work on the Practice Exam included in this book. Do not read the answers to the questions during the time you have set aside to work on the exam - the point is to assess your ability to work under timed conditions.

Do not despair if at the onset of revising you don't understand any of the questions! Things can only get better! Try to do as many MCQs as possible. PasTest publish a number of books which contain MCQs suitable for MRCP Part 1 General Medicine candidates, and since 50% of the questions in the Paediatric exam are on General Medicine subjects these books can help you to identify and iron out any particular weaknesses.

MCQ Exam Technique
There are two common mistakes which cause good candidates to fail the MRCP Part 1. These are failing to read the directions and questions carefully enough, and failing to fill in the computer answer sheet properly.

You must read the question (both stem and items) carefully. Regard each item as being independent of every other item, each refers to a specific quantum of knowledge. The item (or the stem and the item taken together) make up a statement. You are required to indicate whether you regard this statement as "True" or "False", and you are also able to indicate that you "Don't Know". A system of negative marking is used. For every correct answer you gain a mark (+1) and for every incorrect answer you lose a mark (-1). No marks are awarded for indicating "Don't Know".

Look only at each single statement when answering, and disregard all the other parts of the question. They have nothing to do with the item you are concentrating on.

The answer sheet is read by an automatic document reader, which transfers the information it reads to a computer. It is critical that the answer sheet is filled in clearly and accurately using the pencils provided. Failure to fill in your name and your examination number correctly could result in rejection of your paper.

You need to decide on your own personal strategy for approaching the paper. Some candidates mark their answers on the computer sheet as they go through the questions, others prefer to make a note of their answers on the question paper, and then reserve time at the end to transfer their answers to the computer sheet. If you choose the first method, there is a chance that you may decide to change your answer after a second reading. If you do change an answer, be sure that your original mark is thoroughly erased. If you choose the second method, make sure that you do allow enough time to transfer your answers methodically onto the computer sheet as rushing at this stage could introduce some costly mistakes.

Some candidates try to calculate their scores as they work through the paper; their theory is that if they reach a certain score they should then be safe in indicating "Don't Know" for any items they have left blank without needing to take the trouble to think out the answers. This is a dangerous game to play, as you cannot be sure of your score. Furthermore, since the exam is based on a pass *rate* rather than a pass *mark*, you cannot be sure of the mark you will need to achieve in order to be included in the top 35% of candidates. A safer rule of thumb is that you will probably need to answer between 230-250 items to gain enough marks to pass.

There are 60 questions to complete in 2½ hours. This works out at 25 minutes for 10 questions. Most candidates fmd that they have more than enough time and there can be a temptation to re-read your answers time and time again until even those that seemed straightforward start to look less convincing. In this situation, first thoughts are usually best. Don't be afraid to leave the examination room once you are satisfied with your answers.

To guess or not to guess
Tests carried out at PasTest's MRCP Part 1 Paediatric and General Medicine intensive revision courses have proved that by far the majority of candidates can improve their marks by making sensible educated guesses. Most candidates fail the exam by a very few marks and becoming a good guesser can give you the extra boost that you need to rise above the average.

Where there is any chance that you can reach the answer by drawing on first principles and your reasoning power, then it is worth making an educated guess.

If you feel that you need to spend more time puzzling over a question, leave it and, if you have time, return to it. Make sure you have collected all the marks you can before you come back to any difficult questions.

If you really have no idea about the answer, then a lucky guess might gain you a mark, but there is an equal chance that you will lose a mark. In this case, do not guess. Use the "Don't Know" option.

Final Advice

Multiple choice questions are not designed to trick you or confuse you, they are designed to test your knowledge of medicine. Accept each question at its face value, do not look for hidden meanings or catches.

The best approach to the exam is to ensure that your knowledge of medicine and its specialties is sound, to answer each exam question to the best of your ability, and to make every possible effort to work out the answers to the more difficult questions.

PASTEST MRCP PART 1 PAEDIATRICS COURSES

PasTest are the leading independent specialists in postgraduate medical education. Over the past 22 years we have helped many thousands of doctors to pass postgraduate medical examinations.

Our popular six-day MRCP Part 1 Paediatric revision courses run three times each year at a convenient central London venue. Each delegate receives detailed course notes consisting of approximately 250 pages of exam-based MCQs with answers and comprehensive notes, plus many explanatory handouts.

PasTest MRCP Part 1 Paediatric courses are
- ✓ Intensive, practical and exam oriented
- ✓ Designed to strengthen exam technique
- ✓ Interactive and entertaining
- ✓ The key to exam success

For full details of the range of PasTest books and courses available for MRCP Part 1 candidates, contact PasTest today:

**PasTest, Dept. M1P, Egerton Court, Parkgate Estate,
Knutsford, Cheshire WA16 8DX
Telephone 01565 755226   Fax 01565 650264**

READING AND REFERENCE BOOKS

General Reference
J O Forfar et al, **Textbook of Paediatrics**, 4th edition, Churchill Livingstone 1992.
V C Vaughan & R E Behrman, **Textbook of Paediatrics**, 14th edition, Saunders 1991.
A D Milner & D Hull, **Hospital Paediatrics**, 2nd edition, Churchill Livingstone 1992.

Anatomy
R H H McMinn, **Last's Anatomy**, 9th edition, Churchill Livingstone 1994.

Child Abuse
R Meadow, **ABC of Child Abuse**, 2nd edition, British Medical Journal 1993.

Clinical Biochemistry
L Whitby et al, **Lecture Notes on Clinical Biochemistry**, 5th edition, Blackwell Scientific 1994.

Clinical Cardiology
S C Jordan & O Scott, **Heart Disease in Paediatrics**, 3rd edition, Butterworth Heinemann 1991.

Developmental Paediatrics
R S Illingworth, **The Normal Child**, 10th edition, Churchill Livingstone 1991.

Embryology
T Sadler, **Langman's Medical Embryology**, 7th edition, Williams & Wilkins 1995.

Emergencies
Advanced Life Support Group, **Advanced Paediatric Life Support**, British Medical Journal 1995.

Genetics
H M Kingston, **ABC of Clinical Genetics, 2nd edition**, British Medical Journal 1994.

Neonatology
N R C Robertson, **A Manual of Neonatal Intensive Care**, 3rd edition, Edward Arnold 1993.

Pharmacology
J Ritter et al, **A Textbook of Clinical Pharmacology**, 3rd edition, Edward Arnold 1995.

Physiology
W F Ganong, **Review of Medical Physiology**, 17th edition, Appleton & Lange 1995.

Psychiatry
M E Garralda, **Managing Children with Psychiatric Problems**, British Medical Journal 1993.

Statistics
T Swinscow, **Statistics at Square One**, 9th edition, British Medical Association 1995.

ANATOMY

Indicate your answers with a tick or cross (true or false) in the boxes before checking against the correct solutions.

1. **The following are true for cranial nerves:**

   - [ ] A the chorda tympani supplies the posterior taste fibres of the tongue
   - [ ] B the abducens supplies the superior oblique muscle of the eye
   - [ ] C the trigeminal nerve is purely sensory
   - [ ] D the oculomotor nerve has two motor nuclei
   - [ ] E the glossopharyngeal nerve supplies the stylopharyngus muscle

2. **The thoracic part of the oesophagus**

   - [ ] A lies posteriorly to the descending thoracic aorta
   - [ ] B lies laterally to the thoracic duct
   - [ ] C has the azygous veins lying posteriorly to it
   - [ ] D lies posterior to the right recurrent laryngeal nerve
   - [ ] E has the left vagus lying on its anterior surface

3. **The femoral nerve**

   - [ ] A supplies the sensory innervation to the medial aspect of the thigh
   - [ ] B supplies the sartorius muscle
   - [ ] C supplies the peroneal muscles
   - [ ] D arises from L4, L5, S1, S2, S3
   - [ ] E becomes the inguinal nerve beyond the inguinal ligament

4. **The following are anterolateral relations of the common carotid artery:**

   - [ ] A the anterior jugular vein
   - [ ] B the sympathetic trunk
   - [ ] C the recurrent laryngeal nerve
   - [ ] D the vagus
   - [ ] E the oesophagus

5. The following structures are transmitted through the oesophageal opening in the diaphragm:

☐ A the inferior vena cava
☐ B the thoracic duct
☐ C the aorta
☐ D the azygos vein
☐ E the vagus nerve

6. The following statements are true:

☐ A the right vagus passes anteriorly to the root of the right lung
☐ B the left vagus produces the left recurrent laryngeal nerve which supplies the cricothyroid muscle
☐ C the right phrenic nerve arises from the roots of cervical nerves 2, 3 and 4
☐ D the right phrenic nerve passes anteriorly to the root of the right lung and descends on the surface of the pericardium adjacent to the right atrium
☐ E the sympathetic trunk runs downward on the heads of the ribs

7. These muscles produce the following actions:

☐ A the adductor magnus extends the thigh at the hip joint
☐ B gracilis extends the leg at the knee joint
☐ C iliopsoas, rectus femoris and sartorius produce flexion of the leg at the hip joint
☐ D gastrocnemius flexes the thigh at the hip joint
☐ E soleus is a plantar flexor of the ankle joint

8. These structures lie posteriorly to the internal jugular vein:

☐ A the thoracic duct on the right
☐ B the phrenic nerve
☐ C the first part of the subclavian artery
☐ D the vagus nerve
☐ E the posterior belly of the digastric muscle

ANSWERS AND TEACHING NOTES : ANATOMY

1. **D E**

    The chorda tympani arises from the facial nerve prior to its exit through the stylomastoid foramen. The chorda tympani then joins the lingual branch of the mandibular portion of the trigeminal nerve to supply the anterior two-thirds of the tongue.

    The lateral rectus is supplied by the abducens nerve (6th cranial nerve) and the superior oblique by the trochlear nerve (4th cranial nerve) – best remembered by the formula LR6 SO4.

    The trigeminal nerve has a motor supply to the muscles of mastication, the anterior belly of the digastric, tensor veli palatini, tensor tympani and myelohyoid.

    The oculomotor has a somatic efferent nucleus which is in the grey matter at the level of the superior colluculi and an accessory nucleus (also called the Edinger-Westphal nucleus) which supplies preganglionic fibres to the ciliary ganglion whenceforth run the postganglionic fibres to the constrictor pupillae and ciliary muscles.

    The glossopharyngeal nerve has a sensory supply to the posterior third of the tongue and carries parasympathetic fibres to the otic ganglion via the tympanic plexus and lesser petrosal nerve. The postganglionic fibres continue to supply the parotid gland, being carried in the auriculotemporal division of the mandibular branch of the trigeminal nerve.

2. **C E**
    Relations Of The Oesophagus

    Anterior
    The trachea, the left recurrent laryngeal nerve, the left main bronchus and the pericardium.

    Posterior
    The bodies of the thoracic vertebrae, the azygos veins, the right posterior intercostal arteries and at its lower end, the descending aorta.

    On the right side
    The mediastinal pleura and the terminal part of the azygos vein.

    On the left side
    The left subclavian artery, the aortic arch, the thoracic duct and the mediastinal pleura.

    The vagus nerves leave the pulmonary plexus, the left lies anteriorly on the oesophagus, the right posteriorly.

3. **A B**

    The femoral nerve is a branch of the lumbar plexus, arising from L2, 3 and 4. Emerging from the outer border of the intra-abdominal part of the psoas it passes between the psoas and iliacus, entering the anterior aspect of the thigh lateral to the femoral artery. It divides into an anterior division and a posterior division.

Answers and Teaching Notes: Anatomy

The anterior division has two cutaneous branches, the medial cutaneous nerve of the thigh and the intermediate cutaneous nerve. These nerves supply the skin of the medial and anterior surface of the thigh respectively. There are also two muscular branches which supply the sartorius and pectineus.

The posterior division gives off the saphenous nerve, muscular branches to the quadriceps and a cutaneous branch.

4. A
Relations To The Common Carotid Artery

Anterolaterally
Superficial fascia, sternocleidomastoid, sternohyoid, the superior belly of omohyoid, sternothyroid. The anterior jugular vein, the superior and middle thyroid veins all cross the common carotid.

Posteriorly
The longus colli muscle, the longus capitis, the scalene muscles, the sympathetic trunk and on the left the thoracic duct.

Laterally
The internal jugular vein. Posterolaterally the vagus.

Medially
The pharynx, larynx, trachea and oesophagus with the lobe of the thyroid gland. The inferior thyroid artery and recurrent laryngeal nerve also lie medially.

5. E

The caval opening transmits the inferior vena cava and terminal branches of the right phrenic nerve. The aortic opening transmits the azygos, the thoracic duct and the aorta.

The oesophageal opening transmits the oesophagus, the right and left vagus nerves, the gastric vessels and the lymphatic vessels of the lower third of the oesophagus.

6. D E

The right vagus lies posterolateral to the brachiocephalic artery, then is lateral to the trachea. It then passes posteriorly to the root of the right lung and descends on the posterior aspect of the oesophagus.

The left recurrent laryngeal nerve arises from the left vagus as it crosses the arch of the aorta. The nerve ascends between the trachea and the oesophagus and supplies all the muscles acting on the left vocal cord; the cricothyroid is supplied by the external laryngeal branch of the vagus.

The right phrenic arises from C 3, 4 and 5, initially descending betweeen the superior vena cava and the right brachiocephalic vein. From the inferior aspect of the pericardium it passes on the surface of the inferior vena cava to supply the central part of the diaphragmatic peritoneum.

Answers and Teaching Notes: Anatomy

The thorax sympathetic trunk is in continuation with the cervical and lumbar trunk, being the most lateral structure in the mediastinum.

7. A C E

Adductor magnus does extend the hip at the thigh due to the hamstring portion of this muscle. The adductor portion adducts the thigh at the hip and aids in lateral rotation.

Gracilis arises from the outer aspect of the pubic ramus and ischial ramus and adducts the thigh at the hip. It also flexes the leg at the knee joint.

Iliopsoas, rectus femoris, sartorius and adductor muscles aid in flexing the leg at the hip.

Extension of the hip may be affected by the hamstring muscles and the gluteus maximus. Abduction is performed by adductors minimus and medius with contributions from piriformis and sartorius as well as tensor fasciae latae. Adduction takes place by adductor longus, brevis and by the adductor fibres of adductor magnus, with contributions from gracilis and pectineus.

Lateral rotation of the hip is due to the actions of obturator externus and internus, superior and inferior gamelli, quadriceps femoris and gluteus maximus.

Medial rotation of the hip is due to gluteus minimus, medius and tensor fasciae latae.

Gastrocnemius, plantaris and soleus act in combination as powerful plantar flexors of the ankle joint, providing forward motion in walking by raising the heel and transferring energy onto the base of the tarsals/metatarsals.

8. C

Posterior Relations To The Internal Jugular Vein

The thoracic duct does lie posterior to the internal jugular vein on the *left*. Other structures which are posterior to the internal jugular vein include the transverse processes of the cervical vertebrae, levator scapulae, scalene anterior and medii, the thyrocervical trunk and the first part of the subclavian artery.

Anteriorly lie the platysma, the sternocleidomastoids, parotid salivary glands, the sternohyoid, omohyoid, the sternothryoid, the posterior belly of digastric, the posterior auricular and occipital arteries.

The common carotid artery and vagus lie medially to the internal jugular vein.

PHYSIOLOGY

ENDOCRINE PHYSIOLOGY

1. **Peripheral actions of adrenal glucocorticoids include**

   ☐ A increasing the threshold of sensation
   ☐ B skeletal muscle fatigue when steroid levels are low
   ☐ C increased protein anabolism
   ☐ D stimulation of growth and fibroblast development
   ☐ E hyperactivity in excessive quantities

2. **Corticotrophin releasing factor-releasing neurones are**

   ☐ A stimulated by gamma-amino-butyric acid
   ☐ B inhibited by noradrenaline
   ☐ C inhibited by acetylcholine
   ☐ D stimulated by 5-hydroxytryptamine
   ☐ E inhibited by stress

3. **Examples of glycoprotein hormones are**

   ☐ A TSH
   ☐ B prolactin
   ☐ C GH
   ☐ D ACTH
   ☐ E LH

4. **Actions of glucagon include**

   ☐ A glycogenolysis in the liver
   ☐ B gluconeogenesis in the liver
   ☐ C a negative inotropic effect on the heart
   ☐ D inhibition of catecholamine release
   ☐ E lipolysis in adipose tissue

RENAL PHYSIOLOGY

5. **The following are characteristic features of the forces controlling fluid exchange across the capillary wall:**

☐ A the hydrostatic pressure is constant throughout
☐ B the hydrostatic pressure is most affected by venous pressure
☐ C the hydrostatic pressure and oncotic pressure both control fluid exchange
☐ D the oncotic pressure is completely formed by plasma proteins
☐ E the oncotic pressure is usually quoted as 17 mm Hg

6. **In the proximal tubule**

☐ A 40–50% of filtrate is reabsorbed
☐ B no secretion occurs
☐ C sodium is reabsorbed by an active process
☐ D the amount of glucose filtered is always directly proportional to the plasma glucose concentration
☐ E nephrons vary as to the limit of glucose load they are able to reabsorb

7. **In water homoeostasis of the kidney**

☐ A the countercurrent mechanism leads to the maximum reabsorption of water in the loop of Henlé
☐ B the ascending limb of the loop of Henlé is impermeable to water
☐ C very dilute urine enters the distal tubule
☐ D antidiuretic hormone controls the movement of water throughout the kidney
☐ E antiduretic hormone leads to increased water permeability in the collecting ducts

8. **Aldosterone**

☐ A acts mainly on the proximal tubule
☐ B promotes sodium absorption from colon and gastric glands
☐ C is released in response to hyperkalaemia
☐ D is most commonly released in response to hyponatraemia
☐ E is released in response to changes in effective circulating volume

9. In the renin-angiotensin system

- [ ] A renin is released in response to decreased renal afferent pulse pressure
- [ ] B changes are detected by cells of the juxtaglomerular apparatus in the walls of the efferent arteriole
- [ ] C angiotensin II is an octapeptide
- [ ] D angiotensin converting enzyme acts by cleaving three amino acids from angiotensin I
- [ ] E angiotensin II stimulates thirst

10. Hypokalaemia

- [ ] A potentially causes an abnormal glucose tolerance test
- [ ] B causes vasodilatation
- [ ] C is associated with polyuria and thirst
- [ ] D is commonly found in metabolic acidosis
- [ ] E is rapidly corrected by the kidney

RESPIRATORY PHYSIOLOGY

11. The following conditions move the oxygen dissociation curve to the right:

- [ ] A high levels of HbF
- [ ] B hypothermia
- [ ] C acidosis
- [ ] D low pCO_2
- [ ] E high levels of 2,3 DPG

12. The following questions relate to the laws of chemistry:

- [ ] A according to Fick's law, the rate of transfer of a gas through a tissue is directly proportional to its surface area
- [ ] B according to Fick's law, the rate of transfer of a gas through a tissue is directly proportional to its thickness
- [ ] C Avogadro's law states that equal volumes of different gases at the same temperature contain the same number of molecules
- [ ] D Graham's law states that the rate of diffusion of a gas is proportional to its molecular weight
- [ ] E Pouiselle's law states the resistance of laminar flow in a tube is inversely proportional to the square of its radius

Physiology

13. Increases in continuous positive airway pressure, at physiological levels, in artificial ventilation

- [ ] A lead to increased alveolar closure
- [ ] B cause a decrease in functional residual capacity
- [ ] C increase right to left shunting at an intrapulmonary level
- [ ] D decrease the surface area for gas exchange
- [ ] E can in excess give rise to pneumothoraces

14. The following are true:

- [ ] A in the coronary circulation 80% of blood flow occurs in systole
- [ ] B adrenaline and noradrenaline increase coronary blood flow
- [ ] C in the cerebral circulation, autonomic sympathetic vasoconstriction has the major influence
- [ ] D in the pulmonary circulation hypoxia is a potent vasoconstrictor
- [ ] E in the renal circulation changes in blood pressure in the range 50–180 mm Hg are controlled by the renin-angiotensin system

15. Surfactant

- [ ] A is synthesised by type I pneumocytes
- [ ] B production may be stimulated by testosterone
- [ ] C by virtue of its insoluble polar lipids increases surface tension at the water–air interface in the alveolus
- [ ] D specific proteins are required to protect the phospholipids from denaturing factors such as fibrinogen which may have leaked into the airway
- [ ] E SP-B is a glycoprotein with a molecular weight of 30–36 kiloDaltons that binds to phospholipids and carbohydrate groups in a calcium dependent manner

GASTROENTEROLOGY PHYSIOLOGY

16. The following combinations are correct:

- [ ] A fructose = glucose + glucose
- [ ] B sucrose = fructose + glucose
- [ ] C galactose = glucose + lactose
- [ ] D raffinose = glucose + fructose + galactose
- [ ] E maltose = glucose + galactose

Physiology

17. The following are essential amino acids required by children:

- ☐ A glycine
- ☐ B valine
- ☐ C phenylalanine
- ☐ D tyrosine
- ☐ E ornithine

18. Saliva

- ☐ A hydrolyses polysaccharides
- ☐ B is secreted in different forms
- ☐ C is an isotonic solution
- ☐ D plays a role in fluid intake
- ☐ E enhances the ability to taste foods

19. Gastric juice

- ☐ A is usually pH 1.0
- ☐ B contains pepsinogens which directly hydrolyse protein
- ☐ C contains lipase which has activity against triglycerides
- ☐ D contains gelatinase which liquefies gelatin
- ☐ E contains intrinsic factor secreted by the peptic cells

20. Bile salts

- ☐ A are involved in protein absorption
- ☐ B induce bile flow
- ☐ C increase motility of the colon
- ☐ D cannot regulate their own synthesis
- ☐ E contribute to elimination of cholesterol

21. In the digestion of fat

- [ ] A absorption occurs mainly in the terminal ileum
- [ ] B bile acids are absorbed in the proximal jejunum
- [ ] C triglycerides are eventually broken down to free fatty acids and monoglycerides
- [ ] D chylomicrons enable fat transport through the capillaries
- [ ] E micelles carry fat breakdown products to the absorptive surface of the gut wall

22. Iron

- [ ] A uptake occurs mainly in the terminal ileum
- [ ] B absorption is enhanced by phosphates and phytates
- [ ] C uptake is an energy consuming process
- [ ] D is better absorbed in the ferrous than the ferric form
- [ ] E absorption is enhanced by citrate

23. The liver

- [ ] A synthesises binding proteins
- [ ] B is involved in the transport of immunoglobulins
- [ ] C is important as a site of metabolic conversion
- [ ] D does not metabolise insulin
- [ ] E catabolises thyroid hormones

24. Regarding liver enzymes

- [ ] A aspartate aminotransferase is liver specific
- [ ] B aspartate aminotransferase and alanine aminotransferase usually increase in parallel with hepatocellular injury
- [ ] C raised aspartate and alanine aminotransferase may indicate blunt trauma to the liver
- [ ] D in acute hepatitis the rise in alanine aminotransferase usually exceeds the rise in aspartate aminotransferase
- [ ] E aspartate aminotransferase is often minimally raised above the normal range in patients on sodium valproate

ANSWERS AND TEACHING NOTES : PHYSIOLOGY

1. **A B E**
   Peripheral Actions Of Adrenal Glucocorticoids
   (i) Maintainance of glycogen reserve by gluconeogenesis in the liver.
   (ii) Loss of structural protein and atrophy of skeletal muscle by increased catabolism and decreased anabolism of protein. Further glucocorticoid deficiency leads to rapid fatigue.
   (iii) Increased lipolysis by decreased glucose uptake and increased free fatty acid release, potentiating glycolytic actions of catecholamines and growth hormone.
   (iv) Maintenance of force and contraction of the heart.
   (v) Depression in deficiency and hyperactivity in excess.
   (vi) Decreased speed of axonal conduction and increased rate of synaptic transmission, thus increasing sensation threshold.
   (vii) Inhibition of growth and development of fibroblasts.
   (viii) Maintenance of normal glomerular filtration rate.
   (ix) Inhibition of ACTH secretion.
   (x) Inhibition of inflammation.

2. **B D**
   Corticotrophin releasing factor-releasing neurones are stimulated directly by acetylcholine and indirectly by 5-hydroxytryptamine. They are inhibited by noradrenaline and gamma-amino-butyric acid. Stress, for example from hypoglycaemia, hypoxia, hypotension or haemorrhage, leads to stimulation of the releasing neurones.

3. **A E**
   Glycoprotein Hormones
   i.e. two peptide chains, all containing carbohydrate components.
   TSH   LH   FSH   HCG

   Somatotrophins
   e.g. prolactin and GH

   ACTH-Related Peptides
   e.g. beta-lipotrophin
   beta-MSH (melanocyte stimulating hormone)
   ACTH
   alpha-endorphin
   beta-endorphin

4. **A B E**
   Actions Of Glucagon
   (i) Glycogenolysis and gluconeogenesis in the liver.
   (ii) Lipolysis in adipose tissue.
   (iii) Inhibition of glycogen synthesis in the liver.
   (iv) Stimulation of catecholamine release.
   (v) Stimulation of insulin release from the beta cells of the pancreas.
   (vi) A positive inotropic effect on cardiac muscle.

Answers and Teaching Notes: Physiology

5. **B C**
   At the arterial end of the capillary the hydrostatic pressure is usually 32 mm Hg. It falls gradually to 12 mm Hg at the venous end. The pressure at the arterial end remains fairly constant, being controlled by arteriolar resistance but the venous pressure tends to be more variable.
   The plasma protein osmotic pressure or oncotic pressure within the capillary is commonly quoted as 25 mm Hg. However an estimated 17 mm Hg of this is due to plasma protein alone. The plasma proteins have a net negative charge which leads to an imbalance of diffusable ions (mainly sodium) across the capillary wall, creating a further osmotic pressure of 8 mm Hg giving an overall total of 25 mm Hg.

6. **C E**
   In the proximal tubule 60–70% of the filtrate is reabsorbed. Sodium is reabsorbed by an active process causing much of the oxygen consumption of the kidney. This process enables other substances to be taken up, for example chloride, water, glucose and amino acids. The transport mechanism of sodium uptake is by a Na K ATPase enzyme dependent system.
   The vast majority of glucose is reabsorbed in the proximal tubule. The nephrons do vary as to the load of glucose they can cope with, depending on the renal threshold.
   Secretory processes occur in the proximal tubule, for example of penicillin, chlorthiazide, para-aminohippurate, histamine and thiamine.

7. **B C E**
   The countercurrent mechanism in the loop of Henlé consists of active secretion of sodium chloride from the ascending limb into the descending limb, leading to very dilute urine entering the distal tubule. To ensure this process works well, the ascending limb is impermeable to water. When the kidney operates to conserve water, antidiuretic hormone acts on the collecting ducts, increasing water permeability. A concentrated environment outside the nephron in the renal parenchyma will create a gradient for water to diffuse out of the collecting ducts, allowing preservation of water and concentration of urine.

8. **B C E**
   Aldosterone stimulates sodium reabsorption from the distal convoluted tubule and this is linked to potassium and hydrogen ion secretion. It also promotes reabsorption of sodium from the colon and gastric glands, the ducts of the sweat glands and the salivary glands.
   Small increases in potassium have a direct effect on the adrenal cortex, leading to the increased aldosterone release and accordingly increased tubular secretion of potassium. Hyponatraemia is a relatively unusual condition in day to day homoeostasis. The commonest cause of aldosterone release is in response to changes in the effective circu-

Answers and Teaching Notes: Physiology

lating volume, leading to aldosterone release via the renin-angiotensin system.

9. **A C E**
A decreased effective circulating volume leads to decreased renal afferent arteriole pulse pressure. These changes are detected by the cells of the juxtaglomerular apparatus situated in the walls of the afferent arteriole, which then release renin.

Renin acts on the plasma protein angiotensinogen to cleave off a decapeptide (angiotensin I), which is converted by angiotensin converting enzyme to angiotensin II by removing two further amino acids. Angiotensin II is a potent vasoconstrictor, it acts directly on the adrenal cortex to release aldosterone. It also stimulates thirst.

10. **A C**
The synthesis of liver and muscle glycogen requires potassium, therefore failure to convert glucose to glycogen may lead to an abnormal glucose tolerance test. Hypokalaemia affects vascular tone causing vasoconstriction. Antidiuretic hormone is less effective if hypokalaemia occurs, such that it is no longer possible to concentrate urine, leading to polyuria and thirst.

Metabolic alkalosis is often found in association with hypokalaemia, this may be explained by the hydrogen ion shift intracellularly to increase potassium level. Accordingly there is increased hydrogen ion loss from the distal tubular cells.

ECG changes occur with ST depression, inverted T waves and enlarged U waves. Frequent arrythmias occur.

The kidney poorly conserves potassium, especially in the early stages of hypokalaemia.

11. **C E**
HbF has an increased affinity of haemoglobin for oxygen, which is essential as the blood reaching the placenta carries a lower oxygen concentration. This effect consequently moves the dissociation curve to the left. Conditions in which oxygen is more readily given up to the tissue are acidosis, high temperature, high pCO_2 and high 2,3 DPG. This leads to the oxygen dissociation curve being shifted to the right.

12 **A C**
In Poinselle's law resistance is inversely proportional to the radius to the power of four. Fick's law states that the rate of transfer of a gas through a tissue is inversely proportional to its thickness.

13 **E**
Continuous positive airway pressure (CPAP) decreases alveolar collapse helping to maintain the surface area for gaseous exchange and the

Answers and Teaching Notes: Physiology

functional residual capacity of the lungs. At physiological levels shunting is decreased. In excess, alveolar overdistension may arise with an increased risk of pneumothorax. Similarly excessively raised CPAP causes compression of the capillary network leading to shunting.

14 B D E

Most blood flow through the coronary circulation occurs during diastole. Catecholamines have a postive effect on the contractile force of the myocardium and influence metabolic rates.

In the cerebral circulation local chemical changes are the major players in the regulation of blood flow, with hypercarbia having a greater effect relatively than hypoxia.

Hypoxia is a potent vasoconstrictor, with persistent hypoxia leading to raised pulmonary arterial pressure, right ventricular hypertrophy and eventually cor pumonale.

In the kidney, the renin-angiotensin system plays the main role in maintaining renal blood pressure.

15 D

Surfactant is produced by type 2 pneumocytes and reduces surface tension at the water-air interface in the alveolus.

It is a composite of carbohydrates, lipids and proteins. Lipids comprise 80%, each having a 3 carbon chain backbone. Hydrophilic groups bind to C1 whereas hydrophobic fatty acids are attached to the C2 and C3 chains. Together with surfactant proteins SP-A, B and C a latticework of proteins, lipid and carbohydrate is maintained. Surfactant production is stimulated by glucocorticoids, oestrogen, prolactin, thyroid hormone and growth factors. Its production is inhibited by insulin and testosterone.

Surfactant proteins include A, B and C. SP-A is a glycoprotein which binds lipids and carbohydrates forming macromolecules.

SP-B and C are smaller hydrophobic molecules, 8 and 3 kiloDaltons respectively.

16. B D

Sucrose = fructose + glucose
Lactose = glucose + galactose
Maltose = glucose + glucose
Raffinose = glucose + fructose + galactose

Fructose and galactose are monosaccharides. Galactose and mannose do not occur in free form but usually in combination with another monosaccharide to form a disaccharide.

17. B C

There are **ten essential amino acids** in childhood, namely valine, leucine, isoleucine, threonine, lysine, arginine, histidine, phenylalanine,

15

tryptophan and methionine. These are the amino acids that the body is unable to synthesise and must ingest. Certain inborn errors of metabolism can result in other amino acids becoming essential, for example in phenylketonuria the body is no longer able to convert phenylalanine to tyrosine, thus tyrosine becomes an essential amino acid.

18. **A B D E**
Saliva is secreted in two forms, mucous secretions (secondary to the presence of mucopolysaccharides) and serous secretions containing amylase. Salivary glands may be serous, mucinous or mixed depending on their cell type:
Parotid gland – serous
Buccal gland – mucous
Submandibular gland – mainly serous but overall mixed
Sublingual gland – mainly mucinous but overall mixed.
The concentration of saliva does not exceed two-thirds that of plasma and remains hypotonic by active secretion, the glands being impermeable to water.
By secreting amylase, saliva is able to hydrolyse polysaccharides such as glycogen and starch. In the absence of saliva, dryness of the mouth and pharynx trigger thirst.
Saliva acts as a dissolving agent for foods enabling taste fibres to respond to them in the tongue:
Sweet – anterior surface and tongue tip
Sour – lateral region
Salt – entire surface
Bitter – posterior surface.

19. **C D**
Gastric juice contents, as a whole, function optimally at around pH 5.0. Pepsinogens are released mainly from the peptic cells of the gastric glands, they are initially inactive until mixed with hydrogen chloride. Accordingly the pH drops to 5.0 and further small amounts of pepsin act autocatalytically. The pH optimum for a stable acid environment is 1.8–3.5. Therefore the pepsins are inactivated on reaching the duodenum.
Lipase is also found in gastric juice, acting on triglycerides containing short chain fatty acids. Gelatinase acts to liquefy gelatin.
Intrinsic factor is secreted by the parietal cells, it combines with and protects vitamin B12 as it passes along the small intestine and aids absorption in the ileum.

20. **B C E**
Bile acids are involved in the final stages of digestion and absorption of triglycerides. They induce bile flow during secretion into bile canaliculi as they osmotically attract fluids whilst being transferred. Some

Answers and Teaching Notes: Physiology

acids are able to increase motility of the colon. Bile salts are able to regulate their own synthesis from cholesterol in the hepatocytes. Chenic acid (cholesterol = cholic acid and chenic acid) suppresses hepatic cholesterol synthesis. Bile acid contributes to the membrane for the elimination of cholesterol.

21. **C E**

    Triglycerides are eventually broken down to free fatty acids and monoglycerides, mainly by hydrolysis of pancreatic lipase action. These products are water insoluble, and therefore would normally be absorbed very slowly from the luminal surface. Accordingly micelles are formed which are able to incorporate and maintain products of fat digestion in a dissolved form. Their formation contributes to bile salts. Micelles also contribute to carriage of cholesterol and fat soluble vitamins (A, D and K). This process enables transfer of free fatty acids and monoglycerides to the absorptive surface more rapidly than individual molecules could have been transferred.

    Maximum absorption occurs in the duodenum and proximal jejunum, the intact micelle does not penetrate the luminal membrane. The remaining bile acids continue in the lumen and are absorbed in the distal ileum. Once absorbed the fat products still need to be transferred which is difficult in an aqueous environment. Thus chylomicrons are formed, these coat the triglyceride product with protein, cholesterol and phospholipid. Chylomicrons rarely pass along the capillaries but can penetrate the interstitial lacteals and so pass into the systemic circulation.

22. **D E**

    Iron absorption occurs mainly in the duodenum and upper jejunum. At low concentrations uptake of inorganic iron is at least partially energy dependent, but at high concentrations a nonsaturable, non energy requiring process prevails. Iron absorption is inhibited by the presence of phosphates and phytates. Further, uptake is better in the ferous (bivalent) form as this is more soluble. Citrates and ascorbic acid provide efficient soluble complexes with iron and thus enhance absorption.

23. **A B C E**

    The liver functions as an anabolic, catabolic and storage organ. The **main roles of the liver** are:
    (i) Processing amino acids, carbohydrates, cholesterol, fatty acids and vitamins from the gastrointestinal tract and releasing such metabolites on demand.
    (ii) Production of plasma proteins (albumin, clotting factors and transport proteins) and synthesising modulating proteins to bind with and thus control free levels of calcium, magnesium and drugs.

(iii) Transport of immunoglobulins and clearance of antigens by the Kupffer cells.
(iv) Production of coagulation factors and clearance of activated factors.
(v) Metabolic conversion of endogenous and exogenous compounds.
(vi) Synthesis of bile acids from cholesterol and secretion into the intestine. This is regulated to allow efficient emulsification of dietary fat.
(vii) Catabolism of thyroid and steroid hormones and metabolism of insulin.

24. B C D E
Alanine aminotransferase is liver specific whilst aspartate aminotransferase occurs in the liver and other organs such as muscle. These enzymes usually rise in parallel with acute hepatocellular injury, for example viral hepatitis, toxic injury and Reye's syndrome. Further increases may indicate blunt trauma to the liver. In acute hepatitis the level of alanine aminotransferase tends to be higher than that of aspartate aminotransferase and in metabolic disease the level of aspartate aminotransferase is greater.

Patients on sodium valproate often have slightly raised aspartate aminotransferase, this is not an indication to stop the medication.

BIOCHEMISTRY

1. **Plasmids**

   - [ ] A are composed of extrachromosomal double stranded DNA
   - [ ] B are routinely used to characterise within species types of bacteria and viruses
   - [ ] C can be used to trace nosocomial spread of infection
   - [ ] D can be analysed by electrophoresis with the large particles migrating faster than the smaller plasmids in the gel
   - [ ] E are present within the cellular nucleus

2. **Essential amino acids include**

   - [ ] A glycine
   - [ ] B aspartate
   - [ ] C valine
   - [ ] D leucine
   - [ ] E lecithin

3. **False-positive sweat tests may be seen in**

   - [ ] A ectodermal dysplasia
   - [ ] B hyperthyroidism
   - [ ] C abetalipoproteinaemia
   - [ ] D fucidosis
   - [ ] E nephrogenic diabetes inspidus

4. **At the end of glycolysis each molecule of glucose produces**

   - [ ] A 3 molecules of pyruvate
   - [ ] B 2 molecules of NAD^+
   - [ ] C 2 molecules of hydrogen ion
   - [ ] D 1 molecule of fructose 6 phosphate
   - [ ] E 2 molecules of adenine triphosphate

Biochemistry

5. Insulin

- [ ] A is largely secreted as proinsulin
- [ ] B stimulates glycogenolysis
- [ ] C inhibits lipase stimulating the conversion of triglycerides to glycerol and free fatty acids
- [ ] D if deficient causes an increase in amino acid breakdown from muscle which then enters the gluconeogenesis pathways
- [ ] E overall causes an increased release of glucose from stores

6. The following are components of the urea cycle:

- [ ] A arginosuccinate
- [ ] B beta–2 dehydroxylysine
- [ ] C citrulline
- [ ] D carbamoyl phosphate
- [ ] E ornithine

7. The following are true:

- [ ] A cholesterol is a 4 ring carbon structure
- [ ] B sphingomyelin arises from condensation reactions of lysine and aspartic acid
- [ ] C the conversion of tyrosine to phenylalanine alters tetrahydrobiotin to dihydrobiotin
- [ ] D noradrenaline is broken by monoamine oxidase to 3,4 dihydroxyphenylglycoaldehyde
- [ ] E serotonin is synthesised from tryptophan via an intermediate chemical, 5-hydroxytryptophan

8. The following is true for these DNA manipulative enzymes:

- [ ] A nucleases add chemical groups
- [ ] B ligases cut between base pairs
- [ ] C polymerases cleave nucleotides one at a time from the end of a DNA molecule
- [ ] D endonucleases break internal phosphodiester bonds within a DNA molecule
- [ ] E reverse transcriptase copies DNA molecules over 1 megaDalton

ANSWERS AND TEACHING NOTES : BIOCHEMISTRY

1. **A C**
   Plasmids can be used for examination of within-species variation of bacteria but not viruses. They are composed of extrachromosomal DNA and can be used epidemiologically as well as for infection control purposes. In electrophoresis the smaller particles move faster towards the electrode as they offer less resistance.

2. **C D**
   The essential amino acids are isoleucine, leucine, lysine, methionine, threonine, tryptophan, valine, histidine, phenylalanine and arginine.

3. **A D E**
   Other causes include hypothyroidism, adrenal insufficency, glycogen storage disease type 1, mucopolysaccharidosis, severe malnourishment, pituitary insufficiency and HIV infection.

4. **B C E**
   The stages of glycolysis are

   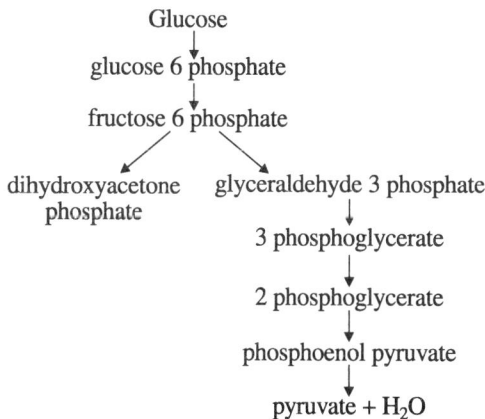

   One molecule of glucose is metabolised to produce 2 molecules of pyruvate, 2 molecules of adenine triphosphate and 2 molecules of *reduced* NADH.
   Dihydroxyacetone is converted to glyceraldehyde–3–phosphate, hence 2 molecules of glyceraldehyde–3–phosphate are metabolised.

5. **D**
   The net **effect of insulin** is to
   (i) increase glucose clearance from the blood by stimulating cellular uptake and increasing glycogenesis
   (ii) decrease glucose release from stores, decrease the breakdown of proteins to amino acids, decrease lipolysis, decrease glycogenesis and gluconeogenesis.

Answers and Teaching Notes: Biochemistry

It antagonises the influences of growth hormone, cortisol, adrenaline and glucagon. All these have the opposing effects to insulin, bar glycogenesis on which these substances have no effect.

6. **A C D E**
Carbon dioxide and ammonium ions combine in the presence of ATP to form carbamoyl phosphate. This reacts with ornithine to form citrulline. Aspartic acid reacts with citrulline to produce arginosuccinate. This reaction is ATP dependent. Arginosuccinate is hydrolysed, liberating arginine and fumarate. Then arginase cleaves urea from arginine producing ornithine, completing the urea cycle.

7. **A D E**
Cholesterol is a 4 fused ring carbon molecule, originally derived from acetyl-CoA.

Sphingomyelin is a cerebroside, a phospholipid synthesized from choline and sphingosine.

Phenylalanine is converted to tyrosine by the oxygenation of tetrahydrobiotin to dihydrobiotin. The failure of conversion of phenylalanine to tyrosine causes phenylketonuria, the commonest cause of which is deficiency of phenylalanine hydroxylase. The deficiency of tetrahydrobiotin is also a recognised cause of this condition.

Noradrenaline is initially broken down by monoamine oxidase to 3,4 dihydroxyphenylglycoaldehyde and by catechol-O-methyltransferase to normetanephrine. The end products of further reactions of these two pathways are 3-methoxy-4-hydroxyphenylglycol (MHPG) or 3-methoxy-4 hydroxymandelic acid, better known as vanilylmandelic acid (VMA).

Serotonin is produced by the action of tryptophan hydroxylase on tryptophan producing 5-hydroxytryptophan which is decarboxylated by 5-hydroxytryptophan decarboxylase to serotonin.

8. **D**
Ligases ligate nucleic acid molecules, polymerases make copies of DNA and smaller fragments, nucleases cut, reduce in size or degrade nucleic acid molecules.

Exonucleases remove nucleic acid molecules one at a time from the end of a DNA molecule and endonucleases break internal phosphodiester bonds within it.

Reverse transcriptase uses RNA as a template and can make complementary DNA from the matching RNA sequence.

PHARMACOLOGY

1. **Phenytoin**

   - [ ] A is well absorbed orally in neonates
   - [ ] B half-life varies widely in all ages
   - [ ] C may be given by the intramuscular route in an emergency
   - [ ] D intoxication can mimic a posterior fossa tumour
   - [ ] E may cause fictitiously low thyroid function tests

2. **In drugs given as a therapeutic trial**

   - [ ] A it is safe to give intravenous pyridoxine to cases of potential deficiency
   - [ ] B diagnosis of pyridoxine deficiency is usually by oral pyridoxine
   - [ ] C the tensilon test often results in muscle pains in positive cases
   - [ ] D oral biotin therapy interferes with assaying levels of biotinidase
   - [ ] E childhood dystonia may respond to L-dopa

3. **Side effects of cyclophosphamide therapy in the management of steroid resistant minimal change glomerulonephritis include**

   - [ ] A obesity
   - [ ] B alopecia
   - [ ] C glucose intolerance
   - [ ] D bone marrow depression
   - [ ] E a significantly increased likelihood of infertility

4. **A 2-year-old boy presents having swallowed his grandfather's hearing aid battery:**

   - [ ] A he should be managed if presenting within 4 hours of ingestion with ipecacuanha
   - [ ] B his parents should be reassured and the child discharged
   - [ ] C this is a medical emergency in all cases
   - [ ] D the condition is potentially life threatening if the battery is lodged in the oesophagus
   - [ ] E an X-ray of his neck at the time of presentation is essential

Pharmacology

5. These drugs can cause harm to breast feeding infants when given to their mother:

- [ ] A   acetazolamide
- [ ] B   warfarin
- [ ] C   high dose aspirin
- [ ] D   carbamazepine
- [ ] E   carbimazole

6. Breast feeding infants with G6PD deficiency are at risk of acute haemolysis if their mothers are taking

- [ ] A   nitrofurantoin
- [ ] B   sulphasalazine
- [ ] C   iodine
- [ ] D   co-trimoxazole
- [ ] E   colchicine

7. These drugs produce the following active metabolites:

- [ ] A   carbamazepine to carbamazepine 10, 11-epoxide
- [ ] B   chloral hydrate to trichloroethanol
- [ ] C   diazepam to oxazepam
- [ ] D   theophylline to caffeine
- [ ] E   gentamycin to gentocholopipic ester

8 Concerning aminoglycosides

- [ ] A   streptomycin binds to ribosomal protein
- [ ] B   gentamicin acts synergistically with penicillin
- [ ] C   resistance to aminoglycosides may occur by plasmid transmission
- [ ] D   they are well absorbed enterally
- [ ] E   their main activity is against Gram-negative organisms

9. The following drugs increase the lower oesophageal sphincter pressure hence lessening the risk of regurgitation and aspiration pneumonitis:

- [ ] A thiopentone
- [ ] B halothane
- [ ] C dopamine
- [ ] D atropine
- [ ] E sodium nitroprusside

10. Malarial chemoprophylaxis

- [ ] A should be started on arrival in the high risk country
- [ ] B in chloroquine resistant areas may include weekly chloroquine with daily proguanil
- [ ] C includes the use of mefloquine to treat pregnant women in chloroquine resistant areas
- [ ] D should be doxycycline in children
- [ ] E on return to the United Kingdom should be continued for 2 weeks

ANSWERS AND TEACHING NOTES : PHARMACOLOGY

1. **B D E**
   Phenytoin is poorly absorbed in neonates, thus the intravenous route is often required to reach therapeutic levels. The intramuscular route should be avoided as it is poorly absorbed and may cause muscle necrosis.
   There is a wide variability in plasma half-lives depending on the age:

Premature infants	10–140 hours
Neonates	10–30 hours
Children and adults	5–30 hours

   Phenytoin overdose or intoxication often mimics a posterior fossa tumour with nystagmus, ataxia, dysarthria and diplopia and may result in encephalopathy with psychosis and increased seizure frequency. Phenytoin is metabolised by the liver, therefore it is a useful drug in children with renal disease. It does have side effects of a morbilliform rash, rarely becoming Stevens-Johnson syndrome. Further hirsuitism, gum hypertrophy and blood dyscrasias secondary to bone marrow toxicity may be seen. There may be fictitiously low thyroid function tests. Megaloblastic anaemia, secondary to folate deficiency and rickets or osteomalacia have been noted in children on phenytoin.

2. **C E**
   Neonatal fitting due to pyridoxine deficiency can be confirmed by a bolus of intravenous pyridoxine (50 mg), preferably whilst an EEG is running. Sensitive cases are confirmed by a resolution in spikes. However this is a hazardous procedure often accompanied by transient apnoea and cardiac arrest, thus it is wise to have full resuscitation equipment available.
   Intravenous edrophonium given in the tensilon test often triggers painful muscle cramps in sensitive cases.
   Biotin assay is still accurate whether the patient is on therapy or not.
   Children who show features of juvenile Parkinson's are occasionally responsive to L-dopa.

3. **B D**
   Side effects of cyclophosphamide therapy include alopecia and bone marrow depression.
   Infertility is unlikely at the dosage used in the treatment of minimal change glomerulonephritis; however parents are counselled about this rare side effect. Obesity and glucose intolerance are associated with steroid usage.

Answers and Teaching Notes: Pharmacology

4. **D E**
   Swallowed button batteries do not usually cause any problems as most enter the stomach and pass through the rest of the bowel within 72 hours intact. Emetics are therefore NOT indicated.

   Complications arise when the batteries become lodged in the oesophagus and may cause pressure necrosis. Chemical irritation and liquefaction of the oesophagus may also occur secondary to electrolyte seepage. Both these are life threatening events and require removal of the battery by emergency endoscopy. The batteries should be revealed on neck or chest X-rays.

5. **B C E**
   Acetazolamide is present in too small an amount to be harmful to the infant as are carbamazepine and warfarin.

   High dose aspirin may give rise to platelet dysfunction and there is a possible risk of Reye's syndrome.

6. **A B D**
   Anti-malarials such as Fansidar (due to sulfadoxine), nitrofurantoin, co-trimoxazole (due to sulphamethoxazole), and sulphonamides may give rise to haemolysis in the infant.

   Taking iodine is an indication to stop breast feeding as it is concentrated in breast milk.

   Colchicine is associated with ototoxicity.

7. **A B C D**
   In the metabolism of drugs, active metabolites may be formed by means of oxidation/reduction reactions or by hydrolysis (Phase 1 reactions) or by conjugation in microsomes in the liver.

8. **A B C E**
   Other aminoglycosides alter the bacterial mRNA and hence cause defective protein production.

9. **None true**
   All of the drugs decrease the lower oesophageal sphincter pressure (LOP) and therefore have an associated increase in risk of developing an aspiration syndrome.

   Other **drugs which decrease the LOP** include
   Ganglion blockers
   Tricyclic antidepressants
   Beta-adrenergic stimulants
   Enflurane
   Opiates

Answers and Teaching Notes: Pharmacology

Drugs which increase the LOP include
Metoclopramide
Domperidone
Cyclizine
Edrophonium
Neostigmine
Histamine
Suxamethonium
Pancuronium
Alpha-adrenergic stimulants
Antacids

10. **B**

Chemoprophylaxis should be commenced 1 week before departure and continued for 4 weeks upon return to the United Kingdom.

Weekly chloroquine with daily proguanil is the recommended treatment in areas of resistance to chloroquine as is a weekly intake of mefloquine. Mefloquine has a lower safety margin than the combination of chloroquine and proguanil. Side effects of mefloquine include dizziness and cerebellar dysfunction, convulsions and severe psychotic events. Mefloquine should not be prescribed in the first trimester of pregnancy.

Doxycycline is used as a second line treatment in the third world but does not have a United Kingdom product licence for use in malaria. It should not be used in children.

Pregnant women are advised to take the chloroquine combination and to supplement this regime with daily folate.

EMBRYOLOGY

1. **In the eye**

   - [ ] A development starts in the tenth week of gestation
   - [ ] B the blood supply is via the hyaloid artery
   - [ ] C the cornea is formed by endoderm
   - [ ] D coloboma of the iris or retina develops because of failure of the choroid fissure to close
   - [ ] E congenital cataracts usually develop after the tenth week of gestation

2. **These statements are true with regard to the skin and hair:**

   - [ ] A the surface layers are derived from mesoderm
   - [ ] B melanocytes originate from the neural crest cells
   - [ ] C new cell production occurs in the germinative layer
   - [ ] D deeper layers of skin are of ectodermal origin
   - [ ] E the fetus is coverd by lanugo hair by 15 weeks' gestation

3. **The central nervous system**

   - [ ] A is of endodermal origin
   - [ ] B appears as a neural plate at around the sixth week of gestation
   - [ ] C the region of the rhombencephalon gives rise to the medulla oblongata
   - [ ] D the region of the rhombencephalon gives rise to the cerebellum and pons
   - [ ] E the region of the diencephalon gives rise to the thalamus and hypothalamus

4. **Concerning the pharyngeal pouches**

   - [ ] A they are of ectodermal origin
   - [ ] B the first gives rise to the thyroid gland
   - [ ] C the first gives rise to the middle ear cavity
   - [ ] D the fourth gives rise to the thymus
   - [ ] E the second gives rise to the parathyroid glands

5. In the respiratory system

☐ A development occurs via an outgrowth of the ventral wall of the foregut
☐ B epithelium of the larynx, trachea, bronchi and alveoli are ectodermal in origin
☐ C the oesophagotracheal septum develops in the eighth week of gestation
☐ D the left lung bud develops into three main bronchi and three main lobes
☐ E maturation of the lungs is completed by an increase in size of the alveoli

6. The following are true:

☐ A the fertilised ovum takes 4–5 days to traverse the Fallopian tubes
☐ B within 30 hours following fertilisation the first cell division occurs
☐ C the morula implants into the uterine wall 6 days after fertilisation
☐ D by day 10 the embryo is producing human chorionic gonadotrophin
☐ E the embryonic mesoderm arises largely from ectodermal proliferation

ANSWERS AND TEACHING NOTES : EMBRYOLOGY

1. **B D**
   Development of the eye usually starts in the fourth week of gestation as a pair of optic vesicles on each side of the forebrain. Surface ectoderm then leads to the formation of the cornea and lens. The blood supply is via the hyaloid artery which later becomes the central retinal artery within the optic nerve. Coloboma are likely to develop if there is failure of closure of the choroid fissure. Congenital cataracts are most likely to form in the sixth week of gestation when lens formation is most active.

2. **B C**
   Superficial layers of the skin and hair, nails and glands are of ectodermal origin. Melanocytes migrate to the epidermis from the neural crest cells. New cells are produced in the germinative layer, with a continuous system of sloughing off via the horny layer. The dermis is the deeper skin layer and is of mesodermal origin. The fetus is covered in lanugo hairs from about 20 weeks' gestation, these are shed around the time of birth.

3. **C D E**
   The central nervous system is of ectodermal origin and appears as a neural plate around the middle of the third week of gestation. The developing brain consists of three vesicles:
   (i) Rhombencephalon – myelencephalon = medulla oblongata
   – metencephalon = cerebellum and pons
   (ii) Mesencephalon or midbrain
   (iii) Diencephalon – posterior part of the forebrain = thalamus and hypothalamus and participates with the formation of the pituitary gland.
   Telencephalon – cerebral hemispheres

4. **C D**
   The pharyngeal arches consist of bars of mesenchymal tissue, separated from each other by pharyngeal pouches and clefts. The endoderm of the pouches gives rise to in subsequent order:
   (i) Middle ear cavity and pharyngotympanic tube
   (ii) Palatine tonsil
   (iii) Parathyroid glands
   (iv) Thymus
   (v) Ultimobranchial bodies – later giving rise to the parafollicular cells.

   The pharyngeal clefts give rise to the external auditory meatus and the thyroid gland originates from the epithelial proliferation in the floor of the tongue, migrating to its level in front of the tracheal rings.

Answers and Teaching Notes: Embryology

5. **A**

 The respiratory system is an outgrowth from the ventral wall of the foregut. The epithelium of the larynx, trachea, bronchi and alveoli is of endodermal origin, the cartilaginous and muscular components arise from mesoderm. The lung buds and the trachea become divided from the foregut in the fourth week by the oesophagotracheal septum. The left lung bud develops two main bronchi and two main lobes, the right lung bud develops three of each. Maturation depends more on the number of respiratory bronchi and alveoli than on an increase in their size.

6. **A B D E**

 Following the first cell division, further divisions occur rapidly in succession producing a rounded ball of cells known as a morula (Latin for mulberry). By the time entry to the uterine cavity is achieved, a fluid-filled space has formed within the collection of cells, causing cells to become pressed to one side, the inner cell mass from which the embryo will develop. This fluid filled ball is known as the blastocyst.

 The blastocyst becomes embedded into the uterine wall by actively secreting a proteolytic enzyme. It also secretes human chorionic gonadotrophin which is measureable in the maternal urine from the 10th day following fertilisation.

 The inner cell form changes to become a bilaminar disc. Each disc develops a fluid filled space, the disc closest to the surface forming the primitive embryonic ectoderm whilst the disc facing inwards to the blastocystic cavity becomes the primitive embryonic endoderm.

 The blastocyst cavity becomes occupied by stroma and cells and is termed the extraembryonic mesenchyme. The embryonic mesenchyme is formed predominantly by proliferation of the ectoderm.

IMMUNOLOGY

1. **Lymphocytic interstitial pneumonitis**

   - [ ] A is commonest in HIV positive children who have been infected by blood products
   - [ ] B carries a very poor prognosis
   - [ ] C leads to unilateral reticulonodular infiltrates on chest X-ray
   - [ ] D occurs in association with clubbing
   - [ ] E may coexist with tuberculosis

2. **Developmentally**

   - [ ] A in the fetus, B cells are initially produced in the liver
   - [ ] B the thymus becomes fully functional at about 12 weeks' gestation
   - [ ] C premature infants do not have the ability to reject skin grafts
   - [ ] D circulating B cells are able to produce all major immunoglobulins from 20 weeks
   - [ ] E the first effective immunoglobulin to be produced is IgG

3. **Interleukin–1**

   - [ ] A is produced only by epithelial cells
   - [ ] B induces production of Tumour Necrosis Factor by macrophages and endothelium
   - [ ] C induces release of GM CSF from T cells
   - [ ] D aids B cell proliferation
   - [ ] E inhibits prostaglandin production

4. **The following features are suggestive of an isolated T cell defect:**

   - [ ] A recurrent oral candidiasis after six months of age
   - [ ] B recurrent bacterial infections
   - [ ] C systemic illness following live vaccination
   - [ ] D hypocalcaemia
   - [ ] E nodular lymphoid hyperplasia

5. **IgA deficiency**

☐ A is an extremely rare finding
☐ B may resolve spontaneously
☐ C can lead to increased respiratory and gastrointestinal infections
☐ D is associated with autoimmune conditions
☐ E is commonly found in association with IgG3 subclass deficiency

6. **Functions of the complement system include**

☐ A neutralisation of viruses by C1 and C4
☐ B stimulation of antibody response by C3a
☐ C solubilisation of immune complexes by C3b
☐ D chemotaxis of neutrophils by C5b
☐ E release of histamine by action of C3a

7. **Hereditary angio-oedema**

☐ A is due to C1 deficiency
☐ B occurs with marked urticaria
☐ C may lead to intense abdominal pain
☐ D on occurring, lasts for 2–3 days
☐ E is worse in the first two years of life

8. **A 4-year-old boy with Wiskott-Aldrich syndrome is likely to have**

☐ A thrombocytosis
☐ B raised IgE levels
☐ C reduced levels of IgG subclass 2 and IgA
☐ D an increased risk of developing B cell lymphoma
☐ E an increased susceptibility to infection

ANSWERS AND TEACHING NOTES : IMMUNOLOGY

1. **D E**
   Lymphocytic interstitial pneumonitis is often asymptomatic in children and generally carries a good prognosis. About 30–50% of children with HIV have been vertically infected; blood products causing infection in children is rare. The condition does represent a progressive chronic lung disease with bilateral reticulonodular infiltrates on chest X-ray and infiltration of small lymphocytes and plasma cells. Gross changes may be visible on chest X-ray with little clinical evidence, although eventually shortness of breath, hypoxia and clubbing are seen. Frequently chest infections, such as tuberculosis, common bacterial and opportunistic infections are seen.

2. **B D**
   In the fetus the liver is initially responsible for the production of T cells. At 7–8 weeks the thymus starts to take over and becomes fully effective by 12 weeks. The fetus can produce all major immunoglobulins by 20 weeks. Accordingly even a premature infant is able to reject a skin graft by mounting a graft versus host response. The first immunoglobulin to be produced, often in response to intrauterine infections is IgM, although adult levels are not reached until one year of age.

3. **B C D**
   Interleukin–1 is released by antigen presenting cells (APC) and thus may be released by a large number of cell types in response to damage, infection or antigens. It acts on T helper cells, aiding the production of lymphokines and particularly interleukin–2 expression. It potentiates proliferation and differentiation of B cells. It aids non-killer cell cytocidal activity, metabolic activation of chemotaxis by polymorphs and increases prostaglandin production by macrophages, again leading to increased cytocidal activity. Further interleukin–1 induces production of TNF from macrophages and endothelium, interleukin–6 from fibroblasts and GM-CSF from T cells.

4. **A C D**
   T cell defects should be suspected when clinical illness occurs following live vaccinations and life threatening illness occurs following usually benign viral infections (e.g. varicella infection). Persistent oral candidiasis after six months of age and persistent mucocutaneous candidiasis are suggestive of T cell deficiency. Certain morphological features tend to occur, for example fine hair, short-limbed dwarfism and cartilage-hair hypoplasia on X-ray. Di George syndrome (with classic cardiac and facial signs) may first present with hypocalcaemia. Graft versus host disease may occur after transfusions, unless the blood is irradiated. Bacterial infection and nodular lymphoid hyperplasia are suggestive of isolated B cell defects.

Answers and Teaching Notes: Immunology

5. **B C D**
   IgA deficiency is a surprisingly common finding in asymptomatic children. Very low levels are associated with an increased incidence of respiratory and gastrointestinal infections and also autoimmune conditions such as SLE and rheumatoid arthritis. Deficiency states may gradually resolve by 3–5 years of age. The reduced levels are often found in association with IgG2 or 4 subclass deficiency, when there may be marked lung involvement.

6. **A C E**
   The complement system participates in various functions of host defence, including C1 and C4 neutralisation of viruses. C3a, C4a and C5a all have the ability to bind to mast cells and leukocytes, triggering the release of histamine and other mediators, leading to vasodilation, swelling and inflammation. C3a leads to suppression, not stimulation, of antibody response and C3b can enhance cell-mediated cytotoxity and solubilisation of immune complexes. C5b can enhance antibody response and lead to chemotaxis of neutrophils, monocytes and eosinophils.

7. **C D**
   This inherited condition is due to deficiency of C1 inhibitor which allows excessive stimulation of C2 and C4 and accordingly release of vasoactive peptides. As a result affected parts rapidly become swollen. There is no urticaria or inflammation, and pain is not usually marked except with intestinal wall swelling which can cause abdominal cramps. Laryngeal oedema can cause fatal obstruction. Attacks usually gradually resolve after 2–3 days. The condition tends not to be severe until late childhood or adolescence.

8. **B D E**
   Wiskott-Aldrich syndrome is an X-linked recessive disorder comprising eczema, bloody diarrhoea, reduced platelet volume and increased susceptibility to infection. There is also an increased risk of malignancy.
   IgE levels are usually high and there is an increased incidence of food allergies particularly to milk.

NUTRITION

1. The following are recommended daily requirements for a 1-month-old child per kilogram of body weight:

   - [ ] A Fluids   150–180 ml orally
   - [ ] B Calories   90–115 kcal
   - [ ] C Sodium   1.25–2.5 mmol
   - [ ] D Protein   2.2–3.5 g
   - [ ] E Potassium   2.0–3.5 mmol

2. Human milk contains per 100 ml

   - [ ] A 60–75 kcal
   - [ ] B 8–10 g of protein
   - [ ] C 0.1–0.5 g of fat
   - [ ] D 0.1–0.5 g of carbohydrate
   - [ ] E 1.0–1.5 mmol of calcium

3. The following are recognised dietary requirements for differing ages:

   - [ ] A 500 kcal/day for a 2 year old
   - [ ] B 2700 kcal/day for a 7 year old
   - [ ] C 12.7 g/day protein for a 5 month old
   - [ ] D 28 g/day protein for a 10 year old boy
   - [ ] E 6 g/day protein for a 14 year old boy

4. The following vitamins are fat soluble:

   - [ ] A vitamin B2
   - [ ] B vitamin B6
   - [ ] C vitamin C
   - [ ] D vitamin D
   - [ ] E vitamin K

Nutrition

5. These amino acid disorders may respond to the administration of the following:

- [ ] A maple syrup urine disease with vitamin C
- [ ] B homocystinuria with vitamin B12
- [ ] C propionic acidaemia with folic acid
- [ ] D Hartnup's disease with niacin
- [ ] E neonatal tyrosinaemia with vitamin E

ANSWERS AND TEACHING NOTES : NUTRITION

1. A B C D E

2. A E
   100 ml of milk contains:
Protein	3.2 g	(13.1 kcal)
Fat	3.8 g	(35.3 kcal)
Carbohydrate	4.8 g	(18 kcal)

   Total energy = 66.4 kcal (1 kcal = 4.2 kJ)

3. C D
   Protein requirement (g/day) by age:
0–3 months	12.5
4–6 months	12.7
7–9 months	13.7
10–12 months	14.9
1–3 years	14.5
4–6 years	19.7
7–10 years	28.3
Males 11–14 years	42.1
Females 11–14 years	41.2

   Energy requirement (kcal/day) by age:
1–3 years	1300
4–6	1700
7–10	2400
11–14	2700
15–18	2800

4. D E
   Vitamin B2 (riboflavin) is water soluble, destroyed by light and is involved in oxidation-reduction. It is found within animal products, green vegetables, milk and yeast. Deficiency is confirmed by erythrocyte glutathione reductase after adding flavine adenine dinucleotide.

   Vitamin B6 (pyridoxine) is water soluble, destroyed by light and it has a role in transamination, the conversion of tryptophan to nicotinic acid and synthesis of delta-aminolaevulinic acid. Deficiency is rare but may be associated with fits.

   Vitamin C (ascorbic acid) is water soluble, being found in vegetables and fruit. It is easily oxidised, and destroyed by heat. It has a role in collagen synthesis hence deficiency is associated with scurvy.

   Vitamin D is fat soluble. A small amount of vitamin D arises from UV irradiation of 7-dehydrocholesterol in skin; the majority being obtained from food, e.g. eggs, fish. Deficiency is associated with rickets.

   Vitamin K is fat-soluble. It is found in leafy green vegetables and is involved with the production of factors II, VII, IX and X in the liver. Deficiency is associated with haemorrhagic disease of the newborn.

5. **D**

Pyridoxine has been used for homocystinuria and hyperoxaluria.

B12 has been used to good effect in methylmalonic acidaemia and biotin in propionic acidaemia and betamethylcrotonylglycuria. Thiamine has been found to be active in treating maple syrup urine disease.

EAR, NOSE AND THROAT

1. **The following bacteria are commonly implicated in acute otitis media:**

   - [ ] A *Haemophilus influenzae*
   - [ ] B *Streptococcus pneumoniae*
   - [ ] C *Staphylococcus epidermidis*
   - [ ] D *Mycoplasma pneumoniae*
   - [ ] E *Ecchinococcus granulosus*

2. **Complications of tracheostomy include**

   - [ ] A an increased incidence of chest infection
   - [ ] B an increased incidence of behavioural problems
   - [ ] C the development of laryngeal granulations
   - [ ] D haemorrhage from ulceration of the brachiocephalic artery
   - [ ] E the development of a peripheral arthropathy

3. **Indications for adenotonsillectomy include**

   - [ ] A parental concern
   - [ ] B proven obstructive sleep apnoea
   - [ ] C documented frequent episodes of tonsillitis resulting in failure to thrive
   - [ ] D tonsillar hypertrophy
   - [ ] E recurrent otitis media with consequent hearing deficit

4. **A left sided facial paralysis**

   - [ ] A may be due to trauma in the newborn
   - [ ] B may be seen in Goldenhaar's syndrome
   - [ ] C can be seen with eczema herpeticum
   - [ ] D may be associated with chronic otitis media
   - [ ] E occurs in 95% of patients with an acoustic neuroma

ENT

5. The following is true for a midline congenital extranasal mass:

- [ ] A glioma may transilluminate
- [ ] B dermoid cysts are pulsatile
- [ ] C polyps are associated with sinusitis
- [ ] D encephalocoeles are solid but are not associated with a cranial defect
- [ ] E craniopharyngioma may present in this fashion

ANSWERS AND TEACHING NOTES : EAR, NOSE AND THROAT

1. **A B D**
   Staphylococcus aureus not *epidermidis* is associated with acute otitis media. *Ecchinococcus granulosus* is also known as the dog tapeworm and does not commonly reach the ear!

2. **A C D**
   Obstruction of the tracheostomy may be immediately life-threatening.
   Other complications include granulations and crust formation around the site of the tube, haemorrhage from ulceration and erosion through the brachiocephalic artery as well as an increased incidence of chest infections.
   An inability to communicate may lead to an increased incidence of behavioural problems in association with distortion of body image. The use of a speaking tube should help to overcome such difficulties.

3. **B C**
   Adenotonsillectomy is no longer a commonly performed operation. There are clear guidelines indicating the use of this procedure:
   (i) obstructive sleep apnoea
   (ii) documented recurrent tonsillectomy causing failure to thrive.
   Peritonsillar abscess has also been suggested but current opinion is divided as to whether or not adenotonsillectomy is required.
   Recurrent otitis media with middle ear effusion and deafness indicates the need for adenoidectomy (and/or insertion of grommets) but not adenotonsillectomy.
   Tonsillar hypertrophy is not an indication for surgery as this is a normal feature of the development of the immune system.

4. **A B C D**
   Facial palsies in the newborn may arise as a consequence of pressure on the facial nerve intervaginally or by the direct force exerted by forceps in assisted deliveries.
   Ramsay Hunt syndrome is associated with facial nerve involvement. Herpetic lesions of the ear lobe, otolagia, infiltration of the 8th nerve and the tympani chorda are all features of this condition. There may be a residual hearing loss with an associated post-herpetic neuralgia.
   In chronic otitis media, facial nerve palsies may develop secondarily to pressure effects. Cholesteatoma may also develop which can also cause facial palsies.
   Facial nerve palsies account for 25% of cases of acoustic neuromas. Dystrophica myotonia has also been associated with facial palsies. Other causes include diabetes mellitus, hyperthyroidism and tetanus.

5. **All False**
   Polyps are intranasal but are associated with sinusitis.

Answers and Teaching Notes: ENT

Encephalocoeles are solid and originate from the brain, hence must penetrate bone causing a cranial defect.

	Polyp	Glioma	Encephalocoele	Dermoid
Position Intranasal (I) or Extranasal (E)	I only	I+/−E	I+/−E	I+/−E
Pulsatile	No	No	Yes	No
Trans-illuminable	No	No	Yes	No
Defect in skull	No	Rarely	Yes	Rarely

NEONATOLOGY

1. Apnoea occurring in the neonate

- [ ] A is not a problem if the neonate is on CPAP
- [ ] B is an indication to check blood calcium level
- [ ] C may be due to hypothermia
- [ ] D may be due to an intraventricular bleed
- [ ] E is commoner in the premature infants

2. BCG immunisation

- [ ] A is recommended for neonates whose mothers come from endemic areas
- [ ] B should be given subcutaneously
- [ ] C should be given ensuring no further vaccinations are given in the same arm for 3 months
- [ ] D means that other live vaccines should be avoided for 3 weeks
- [ ] E will protect infants born to mothers with active or open tuberculosis

3. Maternal drug abuse

- [ ] A of marijuana leads to major withdrawal symptoms
- [ ] B of cocaine has a high risk of placental haemorrhage and stillbirth
- [ ] C of methadone leads to early withdrawal in the neonate
- [ ] D is associated with post-term deliveries
- [ ] E of morphine leads to later symptoms of dehydration and seizures

4. Serum alpha-fetoprotein

- [ ] A is measured at 12 weeks' gestation
- [ ] B if normal rules out a neural tube defect
- [ ] C may be raised in twins
- [ ] D is abnormally low in Turner's syndrome
- [ ] E is normal in exomphalos

5. Brachial plexus injuries

- A occur more frequently with shoulder dystocia
- B may lead to unilateral diaphragmatic paralysis
- C can cause a Horner's syndrome
- D most commonly involves C8-T1
- E can lead to Klumpke's paralysis

6. Treatment of patent ductus arteriosus with indomethacin

- A should be first line therapy
- B is safe in renal failure
- C should not be given in the presence of intraventricular haemorrhage
- D should not be given if there is thrombocythaemia
- E should be avoided in jaundiced babies

7. Renal function

- A of neonates born at term reaches adult by one hour of age
- B may be gauged from initial plasma creatinine values
- C of the premature infant is associated with poor sodium concentrating ability
- D efficiently clears aminoglycosides in term neonates
- E may lead to delayed frusemide excretion in the first day of life

8. Hyaline membrane disease

- A is more common in babies of diabetic mothers
- B is due to surfactant deficiency
- C is not seen in term babies
- D occurs most commonly at 12 hours post delivery
- E always requires ventilation

Neonatology

9. **Wilson-Mikitzy syndrome**

    - [ ] A has an acute onset
    - [ ] B is usually seen a few hours after birth of premature babies
    - [ ] C may be complicated by heart failure
    - [ ] D is often seen in infants previously treated for hyaline membrane disease
    - [ ] E has a similar clinical picture to hyaline membrane disease

10. **The following are components of the Apgar score:**

    - [ ] A grimace
    - [ ] B colour
    - [ ] C muscle tone
    - [ ] D heart rate
    - [ ] E respiratory rate

11. **The following drugs are correctly paired with their potential teratogenic effects:**

    - [ ] A alcohol and macrocephaly with congenital heart disease
    - [ ] B phenytoin and meningomyelocoele
    - [ ] C isotretinoic acid and facial abnormalities with pinna defects
    - [ ] D penicillamine and cutis laxis syndrome
    - [ ] E lithium and Ebstein's anomaly

12. **The presenting features of necrotizing enterocolitis include**

    - [ ] A apnoea
    - [ ] B bradycardia
    - [ ] C abdominal distension
    - [ ] D intramural gas on abdominal X-ray
    - [ ] E bloody stools

Neonatology

13. Causes of polyhydramnios include

- ☐ A diabetes
- ☐ B immune hydrops fetalis
- ☐ C multiple gestation
- ☐ D hydrocephaly
- ☐ E trisomy 18

14. The neonate of a mother with systemic lupus erythematosus may demonstrate

- ☐ A polycythaemia
- ☐ B rash
- ☐ C neutropenia
- ☐ D atrial fibrillation
- ☐ E anti-Ro antibodies

15. In the infant of the diabetic mother

- ☐ A the infant's brain size is increased beyond normal
- ☐ B the infant's liver size is increased beyond normal
- ☐ C he/she can be small for gestational age
- ☐ D there is an increased incidence of polycythaemia
- ☐ E he/she has an increased incidence of hypertrophic cardiomyopathy

ANSWERS AND TEACHING NOTES : NEONATOLOGY

1. **B C D E**

   Apnoea is a very worrying occurrence in a neonate or at any age. In babies it suggests the possibility of infection (sepsis, meningitis), electrolyte imbalance (hypoglycaemia, hypocalcaemia), anaemia, intraventricular bleed, cardiac anomalies, over sedation or early onset fitting (for example pyridoxine deficiency). Pneumothorax may also present with sudden apnoea and desaturation.

   Once the above has been completely ruled out it should be remembered that premature babies have immature breathing centres, which is why 'apnoeas of prematurity' can occur. These infants are usually managed with theophylline or caffeine.

   CPAP refers to the continuous positive airway pressure from the ventilator to keep the small airways open, accordingly a baby will still be compromised if it has an apnoea.

2. **A C D**

   BCG is recommended in the neonate if the mother is from an endemic area, is known to be a case of active tuberculosis or is going to take the baby to live in an area with a high incidence of tuberculosis. The vaccination should be given shortly after birth into the intradermal layer of the shoulder tip. At least three weeks should be left before a further live vaccine is given and the arm should not be used for other vaccines for at least three months.

   In cases of mothers with active or open tuberculosis the infants must be immunised with isoniazid-resistant BCG within a few days of birth, additionally they must be started on isoniazid from day one. It is necessary to keep the mother and baby separated until the mother has completed two weeks of antituberculous treatment, ideally this should be just before the baby is born.

3. **B E**

   Maternal drug abuse leads to many neonatal effects. Babies of mothers taking cocaine are at greater risk of placental haemorrhage and stillbirth, also prematurity and intrauterine growth retardation. Withdrawal effects include irritability, tremors, abnormal sleep patterns and poor feeding initially. Microcephaly and cardiac malformations have been described in such infants.

   Opiate abuse (namely heroin, morphine and methadone) leads to prematurity in up to 50% of cases, with severe withdrawal symptoms occuring in the first 24–48 hours. Symptoms in methadone abuse tend to occur up to 14 days after delivery. Later signs are diarrhoea, vomiting, dehydration and seizures.

   Infants often require chlorpromazine during the withdrawal period if irritability is severe or feeding is being affected.

   There is little evidence that marijuana has harmful effects in pregnancy.

Answers and Teaching Notes: Neonatology

4. C

Serum alpha-fetoprotein is usually measured at 16–18 weeks' gestation. It is essential that the pregnancy has been accurately dated. A normal screening would not rule out neural tube defects or any other feature, such as twins, Turner's syndrome or exomphalos, which can all have raised values.

5. A B C E

Brachial plexus injuries occur with traumatic deliveries, leading to marked lateral flexion of the neck or traction of the arms. There may be associated fractured clavicle, phrenic nerve damage or damage to the cervical sympathetic nerves.

An Erb's palsy is the most common injury involving nerve roots C5 and C6, the arm being limp alongside the body and the forearm pronated in a 'waiter's tip' position. There is loss of movement. Klumpke's paralysis (C8 and T1) involves the small muscles of the hand and wrist flexors, causing a 'claw hand'. There may also be loss of sensation and sweating.

6. C E

Patent ductus arteriosus should initially be managed by simple fluid restriction, avoiding hypoxia, maintaining the haemoglobin above 12g/dl and diuretic therapy if necessary. Only if these measures do not help should indomethacin be considered. However it needs to be avoided if the baby has any bleeding disorders, intraventricular haemorrhage, thrombocytopenia, necrotising enterocolitis, marked jaundice or any evidence of poor renal function.

7. C E

At birth, renal blood flow and glomerular filtration rate are low, but rapidly increase over the next three days. Plasma creatinine values taken immediately reflect maternal levels and therefore are of limited use.

Renal tubular function is initially immature with the urine concentrating ability being limited by a reduced osmotic gradient between cortex and medulla, there is also reduced responsiveness to antidiuretic hormone. The term infant conserves sodium efficiently whilst the premature infant has high sodium loss.

Great care must be taken with all medication given to neonates whatever the gestation, for example aminoglycosides and frusemide are poorly excreted especially in preterm infants.

8. A B

Hyaline membrane disease is due to surfactant deficiency, occurring most commonly within the first few hours following birth. It is more common in premature neonates and in infants of diabetic mothers.

Answers and Teaching Notes: Neonatology

Surfactant deficiency causes a decrease in airway compliance and hence collapse of the alveolar spaces producing a ground glass appearance on chest X-ray. Respiratory distress may be minimal requiring only supplemental oxygen such as given in a headbox. More severe respiratory distress may necessitate intubation and ventilation and the administration of exogenous surfactant.

9. **C E**

Wilson-Mikitzy syndrome is a condition occurring mainly in premature infants (rarely at term), consisting of gradually increasing tachypnoea, recession and the development of cyanosis, commonly within the first month of life.

The condition may be extremely severe leading to oxygen requirement and chest X-ray changes as with hyaline membrane disease. Infants either improve over several weeks or may proceed to develop persistent lung disease and possibly cor pulmonale.

10. **A B C D**

The **Apgar score** is a reproducible way of assessing a neonate's condition. The time at which the score is attributed should be noted as scores may alter between 1 minute after birth and 5 minutes after birth, reflecting an overall improvement with an increasing score or deterioration in the case of a declining Apgar score.

The maximum score possible at any time is 10 composed of 5 categories, each scoring 2 as the highest score.

These categories and scores are shown below.

	0	1	2
Heart rate	Absent	<100 per minute	>100 per minute
Respiratory effort	Absent	Weak irregular	Strong cry
Muscle tone	Limp	Some limb flexion	Active motion
Reflex irritability response on suctioning the pharynx	No	Grimace	Cough or cry
Colour	Pale/overall cyanosis	Peripherally blue, centrally pink	Pink all over

Answers and Teaching Notes: Neonatology

11. **B C D E**
Important teratogens include:

Drug	Effect
Alcohol	Fetal alcohol syndrome including microcephaly
Warfarin	Hypoplastic nasal bridge, chrondroplasia puncta
Isotretinoic acid	Facial, ear and cardiovascular abnormalities
Phenytoin	Hypoplastic nails, intrauterine growth retardation, typical facies and may be associated with neural tube defects as it decreases folate levels
Tetracycline	Enamel hypoplasia
Sodium valproate	Neural tube defects

12. **A B C D E**
Necrotizing enterocolitis presents with abdominal distension and bloody stools. There may be a raised white cell count, with neutrophil shift and raised C-reactive protein. Apnoea and bradycardia can also occur. Intramural gas can be seen on abdominal X-ray and extending to outline the porta hepatis.

13. **A B C D E**
Conditions associated with polyhydramnios:

Diabetes
Immune/non-immune hydrops fetalis
Multiple gestation
Trisomy 18
Trisomy 21

Major congenital abnormalities leading to disordered fetal swallowing:

Mechanical causes
Oesophageal, duodenal, jejunal and ileal atresia
Cleft palate

Neurological causes
Anencephaly
Hydrocephaly
Meningomyelocoele

14. **B C E**
Neonates of mothers with SLE may have transient signs which regress over several weeks, secondary to transplacental antibodies causing

haematological abnormalities such as haemolytic anaemia, neutropenia, thrombocytopenia and cardiovascular anomalies such as complete heart block associated with anti-Ro antibodies.

Babies may have a rash typical of discoid lupus, which fades in infancy.

15. B C D E

Infants of diabetic mothers may be macrosomic with much of the increase in mass being due to an excess of adipose tissue. Selective organomegaly is also seen with the liver and heart being relatively enlarged but the brain being of normal size.

Placental function may be affected in the poorly controlled diabetic mother leading to a baby small for gestational age.

Hyaline membrane disease is increased by 5–6 times compared with babies of the normal population.

Hypocalcaemia, hypoglycaemia, polycythaemia, hyperbilirubinaemia and hypertrophic cardiomyopathy are also encountered.

RESPIRATORY DISEASE

1. **Asthma**

   - [ ] A does not occur below one year of age
   - [ ] B must have the clinical sign of wheeze for the diagnosis
   - [ ] C is often exacerbated by viral infection
   - [ ] D may be exacerbated by aspirin
   - [ ] E presenting with a pulse of 120 per minute and a peak flow of 70 litres per minute in a 6 year old represents a mild attack

2. **Bronchiolitis**

   - [ ] A does not occur below one month of age
   - [ ] B may interfere with feeding
   - [ ] C does not recur
   - [ ] D is associated with apnoea
   - [ ] E is most commonly due to bacterial infections

3. **The following are causes of persistent stridor:**

   - [ ] A vascular ring
   - [ ] B subglottic stenosis
   - [ ] C epiglottitis
   - [ ] D diphtheria
   - [ ] E laryngomalacia

4. **The following conditions are associated with upper lobe fibrosis:**

   - [ ] A cystic fibrosis
   - [ ] B sarcoid
   - [ ] C bronchiolitis
   - [ ] D recurrent aspiration
   - [ ] E tuberculosis

5. Pneumothorax

- [ ] A should always be managed with a chest drain
- [ ] B is commoner in Marfan's syndrome
- [ ] C is commoner with high pressure ventilation
- [ ] D can be recurrent
- [ ] E may be induced by coughing

6. The following conditions can lead to lung cyst formation:

- [ ] A adenomatoid lung malformation
- [ ] B whooping cough
- [ ] C *Klebsiella* infection
- [ ] D *Mycoplasma* infection
- [ ] E *Staph. aureus* infection

7. In managing wheeze below one year

- [ ] A no treatment should be given
- [ ] B response to ipratropium bromide is variable
- [ ] C salbutamol can cause reactive bronchospasm
- [ ] D all infants should be given home nebulisers
- [ ] E adjusting the diet may improve the condition

8. Alpha-1-antitrypsin deficiency

- [ ] A always leads to severe lung damage before liver involvement
- [ ] B cases should be strongly counselled against smoking
- [ ] C causing severe liver damage invariably leads to severe lung damage
- [ ] D never recurs in the transplanted lung
- [ ] E leads to cor pulmonale

Respiratory Disease

9. The following are associated with bronchiectasis:

- A Kartagener's syndrome
- B Turner's syndrome
- C Edwards' syndrome
- D hypogammaglobulinaemia
- E Klinefelter's syndrome

10. The following conditions move the oxygen dissociation curve to the right:

- A high levels of HbF
- B hypothermia
- C acidosis
- D low pCO_2
- E high levels of 2,3 DPG

11. Restrictive lung defects are associated with

- A an increase in the residual volume
- B a decrease in the vital capacity
- C a decrease in the FEV1:FVC ratio
- D asthma
- E kyphoscoliosis

12. Idiopathic fibrosing alveolitis

- A leads to an obstructive airway defect
- B commonly presents with tachypnoea
- C has fine inspiratory crackles at the base of both lung fields
- D may be complicated by cor pulmonale
- E has a good prognosis following treatment with steroids

13. Stridor may be due to

- ☐ A subglottic haemangioma
- ☐ B laryngeal cleft
- ☐ C hypercalcaemia
- ☐ D diphtheria
- ☐ E vascular ring

14. Definite indications for tonsillectomy include

- ☐ A two episodes of tonsillitis in six months
- ☐ B obstructive sleep apnoea
- ☐ C peritonsillar abscess
- ☐ D suspected tonsillar malignancy
- ☐ E type IIa hyperlipidaemia

15. Wheezing may be associated with

- ☐ A cystic fibrosis
- ☐ B vascular ring
- ☐ C vitamin A deficiency
- ☐ D obliterative bronchiolitis
- ☐ E inhaled foreign body

ANSWERS AND TEACHING NOTES : RESPIRATORY DISEASE

1. **C D**
    Asthma is an extremely common condition with onset in childhood and generally improving by adolescence. It presents with:
    reversible bronchoconstriction
    mucosal oedema
    bronchial secretions.
    The condition may occur at any age, but is generally diagnosed after one year because of confusion with bronchiolitis in young infants. Clinical signs classically involve polyphonic wheeze but may consist purely of a nocturnal cough. Asthma is known to be exacerbated by viral and bacterial infections, cold weather, excitation and certain drugs, for example beta-blockers, aspirin (prostaglandin inhibitory effect) and tartrazine (in food colourings).
    Any child presenting with poor air entry, unable to mobilise unaided, unable to talk (due to being breathless) with a pulse greater than 100 and a peak flow less than 100 (peak flows are usually only recordable in those over 4) constitutes a medical emergency, requiring immediate resuscitative management.

2. **B D**
    Bronchiolitis is a common respiratory infection usually due to respiratory syncytial virus, occurring most commonly below one year of age. It can recur as infants do not become immune. Secondary bacterial infections may occur but the primary infection is viral. Older infants usually cope well with the condition having mild wheeze, minor interference with feeds and being slightly miserable. However premature babies and infants of less than six weeks can be severely compromised with major interference with feeding (due to being breathless and having a splinted diaphragm). Apnoeas occur and babies occasionally need ventilatory support. Infants presenting with bronchiolitis and any respiratory risk factors should be admitted to hospital until stable.

3. **A B E**

Persistent causes of stridor	*Acute causes of stridor*
laryngomalacia	acute laryngotracheobronchitis
subglottic stenosis	acute epiglottitis
vocal cord palsy	foreign body or inhaled hot gases
vascular ring	acute angioneurotic oedema
laryngeal web/cleft	diphtheria
cysts of the posterior tongue	expanding mediastinal mass
cysts of the aryepiglottic folds	

4. **A B E**

Mainly upper lobe fibrosis	*Mainly lower lobe fibrosis*
tuberculosis	bronchiectasis
sarcoidosis	aspiration

Answers and Teaching Notes: Respiratory Disease

histiocytosis X
ankylosing spondylitis
cystic fibrosis

pulmonary haemosiderosis
idiopathic pulmonary fibrosis

5. **B C D E**
   Pneumothoraces vary in size from minimal lung collapse to complete decompression, accordingly children vary with the degree of resultant compromise. A well child with a small collapse can be managed as the air will be resorbed. Clearly larger decompressions in a compromised child require aggressive treatment with chest drain and occasional suction support. Some children also need ventilation for a limited time. Tall slim individuals with a narrow anterior/posterior diameter (as in Marfan's syndrome) have an increased incidence of spontaneous pneumothoraces. The problem can be recurrent and in some cases more likely to recur. Acute collapse of the lung can occur with severe coughing and resultant air trapping as in whooping cough and asthma. In premature babies with chronic lung damage and cyst formation, sudden pneumothoraces (occasionally bilateral) are more likely to occur, especially in the presence of high pressure ventilation.

6. **B C E**
   Congenital adenomatoid lung malformation is a disorder in which babies are born with an area of the lung full of multiple cysts and resultant limited lung function. Infective causes such as *Bordetella pertussis*, *Klebsiella* and *Staph. aureus* lead to abscess and cyst formation in some serious situations. In immunocompromised children aspergillosis can also cause infective cysts. *Mycoplasma* causes more generalised damage.

7. **B C E**
   Recurrent wheeze is a very common problem in infants. Children who are completely well and not compromised can be conservatively managed. However if breathing, sleep or feeding are being interfered with and there is understandably a high level of parental anxiety, attempts to control the situation should be made. Initial review of potential underlying causes such as foreign body, cows' milk intolerance and minor viral illnesses should be carried out. There is no perfect cure for infantile wheeze but in severe cases ipratropium bromide nebulisers may help and salbutamol with care as bronchospasm may occur. More minor cases may respond to simple inhalers via 'a coffee cup' or mask (if the child will comply). Very few cases require home nebulisers.

8. **B E**
   In childhood, alpha-1-antitrypsin deficiency usually causes predominantly liver complications. Only in the severely affected cases with very low levels (i.e. homozygous PiZZ) would early lung damage

Answers and Teaching Notes: Respiratory Disease

be seen. No definite parallel can be predicted by the varying involvement of the liver and the lung. It is essential to counsel children to avoid toxic exposure as would occur with industrial fumes and cigarette smoke. Unfortunately changes do recur in the transplanted lungs and death can be due to cor pulmonale. Current research is investigating the effectiveness of replacement therapy via nebulised alpha-1-antitrypsin.

9. **A D E**
   The following conditions are associated with bronchiectasis:
   cystic fibrosis
   Kartagener's syndrome
   hypogammaglobulinaemia
   Macleod syndrome
   and more rarely
   Klinefelter's syndrome
   Gardner's syndrome.

10. **C E**
    High levels of HbF lead to increased affinity of haemoglobin for oxygen, which is essential as the blood reaching the placenta carries a lower oxygen concentration that needs to be efficiently taken up. This effect consequently moves the dissociation curve to the left. Conditions in which oxygen is more readily given up to the tissue are acidosis, high temperature, high pCO_2 and high 2,3 DPG. This leads to the oxygen dissociation curve being shifted to the right.

11. **B E**
    Restrictive lung defects have reduced residual volume, vital capacity and total lung capacity. The FEV1:FVC ratio is normal or raised. Kyphoscoliosis leads to restrictive defects. Obstructive defects have an increased residual volume, FEV1:FVC ratio that decreases and a decreased vital capacity.

12. **B C D**
    Idiopathic fibrosing alveolitis (Hannan Rich syndrome) is a restrictive lung defect initially recognised in adults but now known to occur rarely in children. Onset is usually noted with tachypnoea, progressing to become present at rest. There is a gradual onset of anorexia, weight loss and lethargy.
    The condition carries a poor prognosis with steroid treatment offering only limited symptomatic relief.
    In the end stage of this disease cyanosis and clubbing develop. Death is due to cor pulmonale and respiratory failure.

Answers and Teaching Notes: Respiratory Disease

13. **A B D E**
    Other **causes of stridor** include:
    laryngomalacia
    acute epiglottis
    laryngotracheitis
    subglottic stenosis
    laryngeal web/cleft
    angioneurotic oedema/anaphylaxis
    mediastinal tear
    papillomata

14. **B C D**
    Relative indications for tonsillectomy include severe recurrent tonsillitis affecting schooling/development and also failure to thrive.
    Tonsillectomy and adenoidectomy are advocated for sleep apnoea defined as at least 30 episodes of 10 seconds plus durations of apnoea in a 7 hour period. Advanced cases if left untreated may progress to develop cor pulmonale.

15. **A B D E**
    Other **causes of wheezing** include:
    acute viral bronchiolitis
    aspiration syndrome
    cystic fibrosis
    immune deficiency
    enlarged paratracheal glands
    tracheomalacia
    congenital lobar emphysema
    left ventricular heart failure.

HAEMATOLOGY

1. Serum iron is often raised in the following conditions:

   - [ ] A anaemia of chronic disorders
   - [ ] B beta thalassaemia
   - [ ] C iron deficiency anaemia
   - [ ] D sideroblastic anaemia
   - [ ] E congenital spherocytosis

2. Homozygous beta thalassaemia

   - [ ] A arises from alterations in the beta globin gene on chromosome 10
   - [ ] B may present with failure to thrive
   - [ ] C is associated with an elevated haemoglobin in infancy and older children *foetal*
   - [ ] D may require desferroxamine treatment
   - [ ] E does not respond to iron treatment despite microcytic indices

3. These inborn errors have successfully been treated by bone marrow transplantation:

   - [ ] A cystic fibrosis
   - [ ] B Hurler's syndrome
   - [ ] C Gaucher's disease
   - [ ] D Fanconi's syndrome
   - [ ] E Chediak-Higashi disease

4. A 5-year-old child is found to have a neutrophil count of $51 \times 10^9/1$. This may be due to

   - [ ] A acute liver failure
   - [ ] B corticosteroid administration
   - [ ] C brucellosis
   - [ ] D aplastic anaemia
   - [ ] E hypersplenism

Haematology

5. Atypical mononuclear cells are seen with

   - ☐ A toxoplasmosis
   - ☐ B herpes simplex
   - ☐ C rubella
   - ☐ D cytomegalovirus
   - ☐ E Epstein-Barr virus

6. The following can cause an eosinophilia:

   - ☐ A penicillin
   - ☐ B hydrallazine
   - ☐ C polyarteritis nodosa
   - ☐ D pneumocystis carinii
   - ☐ E atopic dermatitis

7. These statements are true:

   - ☐ A methaemoglobinaemia is caused by oxidation of copper 2^+ to copper 3^+ form
   - ☐ B methaemoglobinaemia may be due to HbC, an abnormal haemoglobin
   - ☐ C methaemoglobin reductase maintains haemoglobin in its reduced state
   - ☐ D NADH is the energy source used in the redox reactions
   - ☐ E production of NADH arises as a consequence of conversion of 1,3 diphosphoglycerate to glyceraldehyde

8. The following conditions present with purpura and normal platelet counts

   - ☐ A Osler-Weber-Rendu syndrome
   - ☐ B Ehlers-Danlos syndrome
   - ☐ C Bernard-Soulier syndrome
   - ☐ D Wiskott-Aldrich syndrome
   - ☐ E scurvy

Haematology

9. The following are components of the intrinsic coagulation pathways

- ☐ A prothrombin
- ☐ B factor XII
- ☐ C factor IX
- ☐ D fibrinogen
- ☐ E factor VII

10. Neonatal thrombocytopenia is a recognised feature of

- ☐ A systemic lupus erythematosus
- ☐ B maternal ingestion of thiazide diuretics
- ☐ C maternal IgM antibodies
- ☐ D in utero infection with toxoplasmosis
- ☐ E shortened forearms

11. In sickle cell disease

- ☐ A dactylitis is a common presentation in infancy
- ☐ B autosplenectomy has generally occurred by the age of 6 months
- ☐ C sickle lung is an indication for exchange transfusion
- ☐ D aplastic crises may arise as a consequence of parvovirus infection
- ☐ E salmonella osteomyelitis occurs

ANSWERS AND TEACHING NOTES : HAEMATOLOGY

1. **B D**
   Serum iron values are low in iron deficiency anaemia and in anaemia of chronic disorders, raised in beta thalassaemia and sideroblastic anaemia and normal in congenital ~~siderocytosis~~. spherocytosis.
   For hypochromic anaemia, the MCV and serum ferritin provide useful clues to the underlying cause.

Condition	MCV	Iron stores	Serum ferritin
Iron deficiency	Reduced	Absent	Reduced
Anaemia of chronic disorders	Reduced/Normal	Increased/Normal	Increased/Normal
Sideroblastic anaemia	Reduced/Increased	Increased	Increased
Beta thalassaemia	Reduced	Increased/Normal	Increased

2. **B C D E**
   Beta thalassaemia is one of the commonest inherited disorders, arising from mutations (rarely due to deletions) in the beta globulin gene on chromosome 11.
   Presentation may be with failure to thrive, feeding difficulties, abdominal distension with splenomegaly and anaemia. Heart failure is also encountered.
   Laboratory investigations reveal a hypochromic, microcytic anaemia with haemoglobin electrophoresis showing an absence of haemoglobin adult A, an elevated haemoglobin fetal F and varying levels of haemoglobin A2.
   Current recommendations are to maintain a haemoglobin between 12–12.5 g/dl and to use desferrioxamine to prevent an excess of iron accumulation.

3. **B C D E**
   The use of immunoprophylaxis and displacement of recipient bone marrow by the donor marrow has made it possible to treat many inborn errors, previously severely disabling or fatal.
   Bone marrow transplantation can be used to replace abnormal host cells or to provide a transferable element to the deficient host.
   Bone marrow transplantation is being used successfully in many conditions:

   Replacing normal cells in:

   Immune disorders
   Variants of SCID
   Late Di George

Answers and Teaching Notes: Haematology

Wiskott-Aldrich
Chronic granulomatous disease
Chediak-Higashi disease
Kostmann syndrome
Autosomal dominant agranulocytosis
Lazy phagocyte syndrome
Cyclic neutropenia

Red cell abnormalities
Diamond-Blackfan
Thalassaemia major
Sickle cell disease
Spherocytosis
Osteopetrosis (marble bone disease)

or have provided a transferable element:
Chronic mucocutaneous candidasis
Hurler's syndrome
Sanfilippo syndrome
Gaucher's syndrome
Fabry's disease
Refsum's disease
Metachromatic leukodystrophy
Wolmans's disease
Fucidosis
Niemann-Pick type B
Fanconi's syndrome

Many more forms of inborn errors are being assessed for this mode of treatment.

4. **A B C**

A low neutrophil count is associated with aplastic anaemia and hypersplenism.

Non-infective causes of a raised neutrophil count:
Chronic myeloid leukaemia
Marrow invasive disease
(eg. leucoerythroblastic anaemia)
Systemic disease
Acute rheumatoid arthritis
Acute glomerulonephritis
Acute liver failure
Acute diabetic ketoacidosis
Haemolysis
Uraemia
Postoperative states
Steroid administration

Answers and Teaching Notes: Haematology

5. **C D E**
In Epstein-Barr virus, there are usually more than 25% atypical mononuclear cells. In all the other viral infections, usually less than 25% of the cells seen are atypical.
   With Epstein-Barr infection or infectious mononucleosis there is often a leucocytosis seen in the febrile phase with an initial neutrophilia which changes to an excess of mononuclear cells within 7 days.
   Bone marrow studies of infectious mononucleosis show a myeloid hyperplasia.

6. **A B C D E**
Drugs which can cause an eosinophilia include penicillin and its derivatives, cephalosporins, nitrofurantoin, phenytoin and hydrallazine.
   Other pathological conditions associated with eosinophilia are haematological disorders such as chronic myeloid leukaemia, Hodgkin's disease, Wiskott-Aldrich syndrome, post-splenectomy infections due to *Pneumocystis carinii*, dermatological disorders such as atopic dermatitis and dermatitis herpetiformis, and connective tissue disease notably with juvenile rheumatoid arthritis and polyarteritis nodosa.

7. **C D**
Methaemoglobinaemia arises as a consequence of oxidation of the ferrous into the ferric state. This may be due to an enzyme deficiency such as methaemoglobin reductase or to a structural abnormality of the haemoglobin molecule as in HbM which can have an autosomal dominant inheritance.
   NADH plays an important role in the redox reaction and in turn is produced as a product of the Ebden-Meyerhof pathway.

$$\text{Glyceraldehyde} \xrightarrow{\text{NAD} \longrightarrow \text{NADH}} \text{1, 3 Diphosphoglycerate}$$

8. **A B E**
Osler-Weber-Rendu syndrome is an autosomal dominantly inherited condition which is associated with microvascular swelling and fragile new vessel formation. These vessels may bleed, often causing epitaxes and gastrointestinal blood loss.
   Ehlers-Danlos syndrome is associated with abnormal elastin tissue owing to a disorder of fibronectin production. This leads to excessive bleeding and poor wound healing with extensive scar formation.
   Bernard-Soulier syndrome is an autosomal recessively inherited disorder associated with giant platelets and a moderate bleeding tendency. This is due to a deficiency of platelet membrane glycoprotein Ib.

Answers and Teaching Notes: Haematology

9. B C

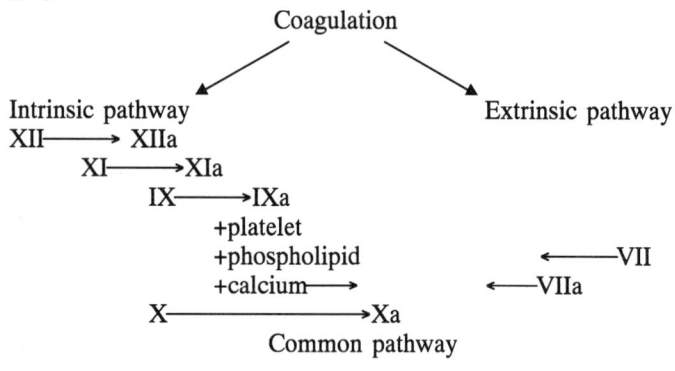

```
                    Coagulation
                   ╱          ╲
        Intrinsic pathway      Extrinsic pathway
        XII ──→ XIIa
           XI ──→ XIa
              IX ──→ IXa
                 +platelet
                 +phospholipid             ←────── VII
                 +calcium ──→        ←── VIIa
              X ──────────→ Xa
                 Common pathway
```

10. A D E

Maternal IgG antibodies are associated with transplacental transfer.

In utero infection may also cause thrombocytopenia, with agents such as toxoplasmosis and cytomegalovirus.

Maternal causes include immune thrombocytopenia, systemic lupus erythematosus and drugs.

TAR is a syndrome of absent radius (this may vary in manifestation of severity) and a low platelet count. The mortality is high initially with 35% of children dying from haemorrhage in the first year of life.

11. A C D E

Sickle cell disease is caused by substitution of valine for glutamine in position 6 of the beta chain in the adult haemoglobin molecule that is HbA, becoming known as HbSS as both beta chains are affected. In heterozygous carriage only one of the beta chains is affected, the disorder being transmitted in an autosomal recessive manner.

There is a high mortality due to an increased incidence of infection, particularly with organisms such as *Pneumococcus*, *Haemophilus* and *Salmonella* which may cause septicaemia, osteomyelitis or meningitis. Infarction and ischaemia may occur affecting organs, bones and soft tissues with dactylitis being commonly seen in infancy. Sequestration crises with splenic, hepatic or lung involvement may be seen and are indications for exchange transfusion in combination with supportive treatment.

Splenic dysfunction is commonly seen. The majority of children will have autosplenectomised by the age of 5–6 years hence the need for daily antibiotic prophylaxis from the time the diagnosis is made. Aplastic crises with a reticulocytopenia occur following infection with parvoviral infection.

ONCOLOGY

1. **Hepatoblastoma**

   - A is more common in girls
   - B may be associated with precocious puberty
   - C is usually benign
   - D responds well to radiotherapy
   - E may be associated with hemihypertrophy

2. **Neuroblastoma**

   - A is the commonest neonatal malignancy
   - B may cause paraplegia
   - C may present with blue skin lesions in the neonatal period
   - D is invariably fatal in stage IVS
   - E may cause a leucoerythroblastic anaemia

3. **Poor risk factors in acute lymphoblastic leukaemia include**

   - A female sex
   - B 5–8 years of age
   - C normal or hyperploidy of chromosomes of ALL cells
   - D white cell count of $2–10 \times 10^9/l$
   - E normal bone marrow response to treatment within 14 days

4. **The following tumours are associated with the accompanying factors:**

   - A intracerebral lymphoma and Wiskott-Aldrich syndrome
   - B melanoma and tuberous sclerosis
   - C retinal tumours and Von Hippel-Lindau syndrome
   - D acoustic neuroma and monosomy 22
   - E retinoblastoma and 13 q deletion

5. A mass in the mediastinum may be due to

- [ ] A thymoma
- [ ] B neuroblastoma
- [ ] C lymphoma
- [ ] D teratoma
- [ ] E rhabdomyosarcoma botryoides

6. Craniopharyngioma

- [ ] A occurs six times more often in boys than in girls
- [ ] B may obstruct the third ventricle
- [ ] C causes hormonal dysfunction in 80% of cases
- [ ] D can present with nephrogenic diabetes insipidus
- [ ] E may show cystic and solid components on nuclear magnetic resonance scans

7. Long term sequelae arising from the treatment of childhood malignancy include

- [ ] A endocrine dysfunction
- [ ] B infertility
- [ ] C short stature
- [ ] D eczema
- [ ] E cardiomyopathy

8. In Hodgkin's disease

- [ ] A marrow involvement is common at presentation
- [ ] B radiotherapy can be used alone in stage III
- [ ] C lymph node biopsy is necessary to ascertain prognosis
- [ ] D 60% of cases involve the mediastinum
- [ ] E the lymphocyte depleted form has the best prognosis

9. Wilms' tumour

- [ ] A has an incidence of 1 in 1 000 000 live births in the UK
- [ ] B is associated with hypertension in 5–10% of cases
- [ ] C may present with peritionitis
- [ ] D typically metastases to the chest
- [ ] E confined to the abdomen lies within stage 3 classification

ANSWERS AND TEACHING NOTES : ONCOLOGY

1. **B E**
    Hepatoblastomas are primary malignant liver tumours, they are more common in boys and usually present before 2 years of age.
    Presentation is generally with anorexia, weight loss, vomiting and abdominal distension. There may be a palpable abdominal mass.
    Other signs less commonly encountered include precocious puberty, hemihypertrophy and hypercholesterolaemia.
    Serum alpha-fetoprotein is grossly elevated.
    Treatment includes total primary resection followed by chemotherapy. Radiotherapy is not effective.

2. **A B C E**
    Neuroblastomas are the commonest malignancies in the neonatal period occurring in 6/10 000 live births per year. The majority of tumours are intra-abdominal causing a palpable abdominal mass. Thoracic lesions may arise in the posterior mediastinum and cause paraplegia by direct compression on the spinal cord. Horner's syndrome may arise in a similar fashion by compression of the recurrrent laryngeal nerve.
    Involvement of the bone medulla may displace a considerable amount of marrow hence a leucoerythroblastic anaemia picture may be seen.
    Stage IV refers to tumours which have spread to involve other soft tissues such as skin, liver or bone marrow but have not caused bony metastases.
    The appearance of bluish cutaneous metastases with hepatic enlargement due to tumour involvement in a neonate is known as the 'blueberry muffin'. The prognosis for this stage is good as spontaneous regression is frequently observed with hypertension from release of catecholamines or respiratory distress arising from the physical compression of the enlarged liver being the recognised complications.

3. **ALL FALSE**
    Poor risk factors include a white cell count greater than $100 \times 10^9/1$, either younger than 1 year or older than 11 years, being male with a normal haemoglobin and low platelet count. Diffuse lymphadenopathy with mediastinal involvement and B cell differentiation on bone marrow are also poor prognostic indicators. Other poor risk factors include an incomplete response to treatment by the bone marrow with cranial involvement or the presence of ALL cells within the CSF.
    Chromosomal analysis of this group often shows translocations within a large number of cells whereas in the good prognosis group, there may be more than 50 chromosomes in these cells (hyperploidy).

4. **A C D E**
    Wiskott-Aldrich syndrome is also associated with ataxia and telangiectasia.
    Tuberous sclerosis is associated with glial ependyomas.

Von Hippel-Lindau syndrome is linked to cerebellar tumours, retinal tumours and to phaeochromocytomas.

Meningomas and acoustic neuromas are seen in monosomy 22, and retinoblastomas and pinealoblastomas with 13 q deletion.

5. **A B C D**
Apart from rhabdomyosarcoma botryoides which is a vaginal tumour all the other tumours may arise in the mediastinum. These may cause airway obstruction, wheeze, cough and dyspnoea. Calcification may be seen in the teratoma owing to the presence of partially or completely developed abnormal mesenchymal tissue such as teeth.

6. **B E**
Signs seen in craniopharyngoma include optic disc pallor owing to optic atrophy, occasionally papilloedema from raised intracranial pressure (obstruction of the third ventricle and compression of the foramen of Monro are also seen), and visual disturbances owing to pressure on the optic chiasma. Pressure on the pituitary/hypothalamic axis can lead to deficiencies in growth hormone, thyroid stimulating hormone, antidiuretic hormone and adrenocorticotrophic hormone. Presentation therefore may be with short stature or other abnormal endocrine disorders.

7. **A B C E**
Chemotherapy has caused iatrogenic disorders for example cardiomyopathy has been seen following treatment with doxorubicin.

Cranial irradiation may cause endocrine dysfunction and short stature. Radiation in other sites has also given rise to pulmonary fibrosis, hepatitis and enteritis with scoliosis and other vertebral defects. These complications may have arisen as a consequence of previously higher doses of radiation having been used.

Other complications following treatment of primary malignancy include recurrence, the development of another type of malignancy and damage to other organs consequent to the type of treatments used. Educational and psychological problems may also arise, for example difficulties with obtaining employment and getting insurance policies owing to the previous medical history.

8. **C D**
There are four **histological types of Hodgkin's disease**:

   I   Lymphocyte predominant (best prognosis)

   II Nodular sclerosis

   III Mixed cellularity

   IV Lymphocyte depleted (worst prognosis)

Answers and Teaching Notes: Oncology

Staging depends on the absence or presence of systemic features. 60% of cases involve the mediastinum. Hodgkin's disease commonly presents with cervical lymphadenopathy. Lymph node biopsy is necessary to ascertain histology.

9. **B C D E**
   The incidence of Wilms' tumour (nephroblastoma) is 1 in 10 000 live births with an equal sex ratio. It is associated with aniridia and can be inherited in an autosomal form in some instances. The peak age of presentation is under the age of 3 years with abdominal distension and a palpable mass in an otherwise well child. There is a low grade fever and/or haematuria in 25% of cases and hypertension is only noted in 5–10% of cases. Occasionally rupture of the mass may occur causing peritonitis.

   Metastases are commonest in the chest, but may also appear in the liver, bones and brain.

   Stage 1 refers to limitation of the tumour to one kidney.

   Stage 2 is seen where there is extension of the tumour to the accompanying renal vessels or the outer capsule of the kidney and perinephric fascia.

   Stage 3 refers to non-haematogenous spread confined to the abdomen.

   Stage 4 is seen with blood-borne metastases to organs such as lung, liver and brain.

   All stages bar stage 1 require post-operative radiotherapy with chemotherapy.

CARDIOLOGY

1. **The following conditions may give rise to Eisenmenger's syndrome:**

   ☐ A atrioseptal defect
   ☐ B ventriculoseptal defect
   ☐ C patent ductus arteriosus
   ☐ D coarctation of the aorta
   ☐ E hypoplastic left heart syndrome

2. **The following conditions are associated with oligaemic lung fields:**

   ☐ A pulmonary atresia with intact ventricular septum
   ☐ B patent ductus arteriosus
   ☐ C coarctation of the aorta
   ☐ D transposition of the great vessels
   ☐ E Ebstein's anomaly

3. **These are normal values for cardiac catheterisation data in a 5-year-old male:**

   ☐ A saturation of 95% in the right ventricle
   ☐ B saturation of 75% in the left atrium
   ☐ C mean right atrial pressure of 3–5 mm Hg
   ☐ D systolic pressure in the main pulmonary artery of 30 mm Hg
   ☐ E saturation of 70% in the superior vena cava

4. **Common features of benign murmurs include**

   ☐ A an ejection click
   ☐ B variation with posture
   ☐ C decreasing with inspiration
   ☐ D a diastolic rumbling murmur
   ☐ E a thrill

Cardiology

5. These lesions can present with heart failure in the neonatal period

- [ ] A aortic atresia
- [ ] B transposition of the great vessels
- [ ] C Ebstein's anomaly
- [ ] D coarctation of the aorta
- [ ] E atrial septal defect

6. The following drugs taken in pregnancy are commonly associated with the accompanying heart lesion:

- [ ] A amphetamines and transposition of the great vessels
- [ ] B phenytoin and coarctation of the aorta
- [ ] C lithium and atrial septal defect
- [ ] D alcohol and atrial septal defect
- [ ] E oestrogens and tetralogy of Fallot

7. Murmurless cyanotic heart lesions in the neonatal period may be due to

- [ ] A hypoplastic left ventricle
- [ ] B cor triatrium
- [ ] C coarctation of the aorta
- [ ] D pulmonary atresia with ventricular septal defect
- [ ] E endocardial fibroelastosis

8. Major criteria of the Duchet-Jones diagnostic categories for rheumatic fever include

- [ ] A a prolonged PR interval
- [ ] B a raised ASOT titre
- [ ] C a recent episode of scarlet fever
- [ ] D fever
- [ ] E a positive throat swab culture for group A streptococcus

Cardiology

9. A prominent main pulmonary artery is seen on the AP chest X-ray in

- ☐ A pulmonary valvular stenosis
- ☐ B atrial septal defect
- ☐ C pulmonary hypertension
- ☐ D pulmonary atresia
- ☐ E ventricular septal defect

10. A child with central cyanosis and increased pulmonary vascular markings may have

- ☐ A transposition of the great vessels
- ☐ B total anomalous pulmonary venous return
- ☐ C persistent truncus arteriosus
- ☐ D ventricular septal defect
- ☐ E patent ductus arteriosus

11. A child who is cyanosed with decreased pulmonary markings on chest X-ray may have

- ☐ A coarctation of the aorta
- ☐ B mitral stenosis
- ☐ C tricuspid atresia
- ☐ D pulmonary stenosis
- ☐ E tetralogy of Fallot

12. A 3-month-old child is brought to the accident and emergency department unconscious and poorly peripherally perfused. His capillary return is 6 seconds and his heart rate is 240 beats per minute on the ECG monitor with a regular narrow complex appearance. He is intubated and ventilated adequately but still his circulation appears compromised. The most effective immediate treatment is

- ☐ A a vagal manoeuvre
- ☐ B AC shock at 2 J/kg
- ☐ C the use of synchronised DC cardioversion starting at 0.5 J/kg
- ☐ D to give adenosine 0.5 mg/kg intravenously
- ☐ E to stimulate the diving reflex

Cardiology

13. **Aberrant pathways of electrical conduction within the heart are seen with**

   ☐ A myocarditis
   ☐ B Ebstein's anomaly
   ☐ C cardiac tamponade
   ☐ D Wolff-Parkinson-White syndrome
   ☐ E the vein of Galen aneurysm

14. **These conditions are associated with high output cardiac states:**

   ☐ A septic shock
   ☐ B thyrotoxicosis
   ☐ C anaemia
   ☐ D the vein of Galen aneurysm
   ☐ E ulcerative colitis

ANSWERS AND TEACHING NOTES : CARDIOLOGY

1. **A B C**
   Eisenmenger's syndrome arises as a consequence of pulmonary hypertension, with the pulmonary resistance overcoming systemic vascular resistance; this leads to right to left flow. Hence any cardiac lesion in which there is reversed shunting may be termed Eisenmenger's syndrome.
   These lesions include patent ductus arteriosus, ventriculoseptal defects, atrial septal defects, atrioventricular canal defects and aortopulmonary window. More complex heart disease such as persistent truncus arteriosus, transposition of the great vessels with a communication between systemic and pulmonary circulations and total anomalous pulmonary venous drainage can also give rise to Eisenmenger's syndrome.

2. **A E**
   The presence of oligaemic lung fields on chest X-ray indicates a heart lesion with poor pulmonary blood flow.
   Pulmonary atresia with intact septum and Ebstein's anomaly are associated with decreased pulmonary blood flow.

3. **C D E**

	Saturation (%)	Blood pressure (mm Hg)
Inferior vena cava	75	3–5
Superior vena cava	70	3–5
Right atrium	73	3–5
Right ventricle	73	30/5
Main pulmonary artery	73	30/12
Left atrium	95	5–7
Left ventricle	95	100/6
Ascending aorta	95	100/60

   Blood pressure measurements with / indicate systolic and diastolic values, otherwise figures quoted are for mean blood pressure values.

4. **B C**
   Benign or innocent murmurs are common in childhood. They vary with posture and respiration and tend to occur in systole. A thrill or a diastolic murmur is suggestive of structural abnormality.

5. **A D**
   Transposition of the great vessels and Ebstein's anomaly present with cyanosis in the neonatal period.
   Coarctation of the aorta with or without ventricular septal defect(s) may present with heart failure depending on the severity of the stenosis. Other lesions apart from aortic atresia include patent ductus arteriosus. Obstructed total anomalous pulmonary venous drainage tends to present with cyanosis as do pulmonary atresia, critical pulmonary stenosis and severe tricuspid atresia.

Answers and Teaching Notes: Cardiology

6. **A B D E**
   Lithium is commonly associated with Ebstein's anomaly.
   Alcohol and amphetamines are associated with transposition of the great vessels, atrial and ventricular septal defects as well as patent ductus arteriosus.
   Phenytoin is associated with pulmonary and aortic stenosis and patent ductus arteriosus. Oestrogens and progestogens are associated with tetralogy of Fallot, transposition and ventricular septal defects.

7. **A D**
   Lesions which may present in the newborn period with cyanosis but no murmur include transposition of the great arteries, total anomalous pulmonary venous drainage, hypoplastic left ventricle, pulmonary atresia with and without intact ventricular septum, and tricuspid atresia.
   Lesions such as coarctation of the aorta, cor triatrium and endocardial fibroelastosis are acyanotic heart lesions and may not necessarily have a murmur associated with them.

8. **ALL FALSE**

Major criteria	Minor criteria
Polyarthritis	Fever
Carditis	Arthralgia
Sydenham's chorea	Previous history of rheumatic fever
Subcutaneous nodules	Increased inflammatory markers eg raised ESR or CRP
Erythema nodosum	

   Preceding evidence of streptococcal infection includes one of the following: increased ASOT, positive throat swab culture for group A streptococcus, and a recent history of scarlet fever.
   The diagnosis of rheumatic fever requires the confirmation of two major diagnostic criteria or two minor and one major. In both instances there should be preceding evidence of streptococcal infection.

9. **A B C E**
   A prominent main pulmonary artery is seen in the following:
   (i) increased blood flow as in atrial septal defect or ventricular septal defect
   (ii) increased pressure within the pulmonary artery as in pulmonary hypertension
   (iii) in post-stenotic dilatation as in valvular stenosis.

Answers and Teaching Notes: Cardiology

10. **A B C**
    A cyanosed child with increased pulmonary markings on chest X-ray may have:
      transposition of the great vessels
      total anomalous pulmonary venous return
      persistent truncus arteriosus
      single ventricle.

    An acyanotic child may have increased pulmonary markings due to:
      atrial septal defect
      ventricular septal defect
      patent ductus arteriosus
      endocardial cushion defect
      partial anomalous pulmonary venous return.

11. **C D E**
    Cyanosis with decreased pulmonary markings is seen in:
      pulmonary atresia
      tricuspid atresia
      pulmonary valve atresia with hypoplastic right ventricle
      tetralogy of Fallot
      Eisenmenger's syndrome
      Ebstein's anomaly.

12. **C**
    The **emergency management of a child with a supraventricular tachycardia with shock** as evidenced by poor cardiac output and decreased level of consciousness is to first open the airway, ensure adequate ventilation and deal with the circulation in that order of priority. This child should be cardioverted using DC shock starting at 0.5 J/kg, the next dose being increased to 1 J/kg and the third dose being 2 J/kg.

    Vagal manouevres and adenosine are not recommended for routine use in the treatment of life-threatening supraventricular tachycardia.

13. **B D**
    Neither myocarditis nor cardiac tamponade is associated with abnormal pathways. The vein of Galen is an intracranial A-V malformation and may be a cause of heart failure.

    Ebstein's anomaly is associated with aberrant pathways, the commonest form being Wolff-Parkinson-White syndrome. Wolff-Parkinson-White has a characteristic slurring of the P to QRS complex called the delta wave.

14. **A B C D**
    All these apart from ulcerative colitis are causes of a high output state.

RENAL DISEASE

1. **In Berger's nephropathy**

   - A   renal biopsy demonstrates signs of minimal change nephropathy
   - B   there is mainly deposition of IgG
   - C   the plasma C3 levels are reduced
   - D   there is a majority of male cases
   - E   symptoms may recur in the transplanted kidney

2. **Alport syndrome**

   - A   occurs only in males
   - B   is always associated with sensorineural deafness at diagnosis
   - C   is associated with cataracts
   - D   is associated with renal failure in the second to third decade in females
   - E   may be associated with changes in the transplanted kidney

3. **In systemic lupus erythematosus**

   - A   presentation with lupus nephritis is rare in childhood
   - B   the WHO have subdivided types of lupus nephritis into five categories
   - C   diffuse proliferative lupus nephritis is the most severe form to occur
   - D   there is a high incidence in girls under 8 years
   - E   there are reduced levels of C3 and C4

4. **Henoch-Schonlein purpura**

   - A   commonly presents with an urticarial or purpuric rash over the trunk and forearms
   - B   is associated with arthralgia
   - C   has mainly mesangial deposits of IgG
   - D   has a 50% incidence of renal involvement
   - E   classically has a reduced platelet count

5. Haemolytic uraemic syndrome

- [ ] A usually occurs in children between 4 and 8 years of age
- [ ] B is associated with primary viral or bacterial infections
- [ ] C often demonstrates helmet cells on blood film
- [ ] D is associated with a Coombs positive microangiopathic haemolytic anaemia
- [ ] E leads to the neurological manifestation of unusual cheerfulness

6. Nephrotic syndrome is complicated by

- [ ] A increased susceptibility to infections
- [ ] B peritonitis meriting Gram-positive and negative antibiotic cover
- [ ] C the masking of infection
- [ ] D pleural effusions
- [ ] E deficiencies in factors IX, XI and XII of the coagulation cascade

7. In proximal renal tubular acidosis

- [ ] A the proximal tubule is unable to reabsorb bicarbonate
- [ ] B the distal tubule initially compensates well
- [ ] C it is possible to acidify the urine
- [ ] D hypokalaemia is a complication
- [ ] E nephrocalcinosis is a complication

8. Distal renal tubular acidosis may occur secondary to

- [ ] A pyelonephritis
- [ ] B medullary sponge kidney
- [ ] C medullary cystic disease
- [ ] D Ehlers-Danlos syndrome
- [ ] E cystinosis

Renal Disease

9. **Bartter's syndrome**

   - [ ] A is usually of X-linked inheritance
   - [ ] B has raised blood pressure
   - [ ] C is associated with abnormal platelet function
   - [ ] D is a cause of growth failure
   - [ ] E is associated with hypokalaemic metabolic alkalosis

10. **A nine-month-old girl presents to clinic with a proven urinary tract infection**

    - [ ] A she could have had an *E. coli* $\times\ 10^3$ culture growth
    - [ ] B if found to have grade I reflux she will need operative intervention
    - [ ] C antibiotic prophylaxis should be stopped to allow reculture
    - [ ] D she should have an urgent MCUG
    - [ ] E she needs an abdominal ultrasound three months after the diagnosis of a urinary tract infection

11. **Congenital nephrotic syndrome**

    - [ ] A is mainly autosomal dominant
    - [ ] B antenatally produces a raised alpha-fetoprotein
    - [ ] C is more common in Scandinavians than in the British
    - [ ] D infants are often premature with an abnormally large placenta
    - [ ] E infants may be oedematous at birth

12. **Causes of a hypokalaemic metabolic alkalosis include**

    - [ ] A congenital adrenal hyperplasia
    - [ ] B Addison's disease
    - [ ] C renal artery stenosis
    - [ ] D diuretic abuse
    - [ ] E Conn's syndrome

ANSWERS AND TEACHING NOTES : RENAL DISEASE

1. **D E**
   Berger's nephropathy or IgA nephropathy usually presents with gross haematuria or is incidentally found in cases with microscopic haematuria. Most renal biopsies show signs of focal and segmental proliferation with increased matrix. The more severe cases have crescents and scarring.

   There are large amounts of IgA deposition in the mesangium and smaller amounts of IgG, IgM, C3 and properidin. Plasma C3 levels are normal.

   There are twice as many males affected as females. About 20% of cases carry a poor prognosis with raised blood pressure, poor renal function, proteinuria and increasing scarring. There is no effective treatment. The nephropathy commonly recurs in the transplanted kidney.

2. **C E**
   Alport syndrome is an inherited condition in which males are most severely affected. Gradual mesangial proliferation and capillary wall thickening develop, leading to progressive glomerular sclerosis.

   Presentation is often with asymptomatic haematuria. Sensorineural deafness is present in a minority of cases at diagnosis and tends to be progressive. About 10% of cases are associated with eye changes, notably cataracts, keratoconus and spherophakia.

   The pattern of inheritance is not known but males tend to be far more severely affected than females and there is a high spontaneous mutation rate.

   Males usually develop end stage renal failure by the second to third decade of life and anti-glomerular basement membrane nephritis may develop in the transplanted kidney. Females have a normal life span and only very mild hearing loss.

3. **B C E**
   Systemic lupus erythematosus is a multisystem disorder which commonly presents in childhood in the form of lupus nephritis.

   The WHO has subdivided lupus nephritis into five main categories:

   Class 1: lupus nephritis with no histological abnormality.

   Class 2: mesangial lupus nephritis.

   Class 3: focal proliferative lupus nephritis.

   Class 4: diffuse proliferative lupus nephritis – the most common and severe form.

   Class 5: membrane lupus nephritis.

   There is often transformation from one class to another, usually becoming more severe.

Answers and Teaching Notes: Renal Disease

Systemic lupus erythematosus has an increased incidence in adolescent girls. At diagnosis circulating antinuclear antibodies reacting to double-stranded DNA are often found. T and B cell functioning is frequently abnormal and C3 and C4 levels are reduced.

All patients with lupus nephritis should have a renal biopsy.

4. **B D**

Henoch-Schonlein purpura leads to mesangial deposits of IgA, frequently in association with IgG, C3 and fibrin. There may also be deposition along capillary walls.

Presentation is usually with an urticarial or purpuric rash over the buttocks and the lower limbs. The condition is often associated with arthralgia or arthritis and abdominal pain. Renal involvement is found in upto 50% of cases varying from mild to very severe. Evidence of renal involvement is usually noted within one month, but may be noted even later. Effects vary from haematuria with good renal function to severe changes with very poor renal function, heavy proteinuria and a nephrotic syndrome type picture.

There are normal platelet and C3 levels and no antinuclear antibodies in the serum.

The condition usually completely resolves over several months, however microscopic haematuria may be found for more than a year. Severe renal involvement carries a very poor prognosis.

5. **B C**

Haemolytic uraemic syndrome is associated with primary bacterial (eg. *Shigella, Salmonella, E. coli, Strep. pneumoniae*) or viral (eg. Coxsackie, ECHO, influenza, varicella, Epstein-Barr) infections. The underlying damaging factor is due to a release of endotoxin causing harm related to vascular occlusion, especially in the kidney. There is evidence of an abscence of a plasma factor that stimulates endothelial cell prostacyclin production.

Presentation is usually in children under 4 years old. The classical picture is:

Coombs negative microangiopathic haemolytic anaemia
thrombocytopenia
acute renal failure.

Blood film often demonstrates helmet cells, burr cells, fragmented cells, raised white blood cell count and in 90% of cases a reduced platelet count.

The children are classically very miserable and irritable. They may also develop fitting, coma, severe colitis, diabetes mellitus and rhabdomyolysis.

Answers and Teaching Notes: Renal Disease

6. **A B C D E**
Nephrotic syndrome is complicated by an increased susceptibility to infection. Commonly peritonitis, also sepsis, pneumonia, cellulitis and urinary tract infections are noted. The causative bacteria are often *Strep. pneumonia*, however Gram-negative organisms may also be involved, hence the need for wide cover. Further there may be few physical findings of infection. In the remission period all patients must be covered with polyvalent pneumococcal vaccine.

There is increased incidence of arterial and venous thromboses secondary to increased coagulation factors. There is a reduction in the levels of inhibitors of fibrinolysis and of antithrombin III. There are also deficiencies of coagulation factors IX, XI and XII and serum vitamin D levels.

7. **C D**
Proximal renal tubular acidosis is the inability of the proximal tubule to reabsorb bicarbonate efficiently, only about 60% is reabsorbed compared with 80% normally. The distal tubule can only cope with reabsorbing 15% of the filtered load, so bicarbonate loss occurs.

Proximal renal tubular acidosis is usually the more severe form compared with the distal form.

Gradual bicarbonate loss occurs initially until steady state occurs, in other words the amount left to be filtered is small enough for the kidney to cope with.

As the distal acidification mechanism is not affected the kidney is still able to acidify urine.

Larger than normal amounts of sodium bicarbonate arriving at the distal tubule lead to increased sodium reabsorption in exchange for potassium. Hence hypokalaemia develops.

Proximal renal tubular acidosis may occur independently or in association with other conditions. It may be transient or a constant feature, sporadic or inherited.

Nephrocalcinosis is a complication of distal renal tubular acidosis.

8. **A B D**
Secondary causes of renal tubular acidosis

Proximal	*Distal*
Acquired	*Toxins*
heavy metals	lithium
lead	amphotericin B
hyperparathyroidism	
vit D deficiency rickets	*Interstitial nephritis*
	obstruction
Inherited	pyelonephritis
cystinosis	transplant rejection

87

Answers and Teaching Notes: Renal Disease

galactosaemia
hereditary fructose intolerance
tyrosinaemia
Lowe syndrome
medullary cystic disease
Wilson disease

sickle cell nephropathy
lupus nephritis
Ehlers Danlos syndrome
nephrocalcinosis
hepatic cirrhosis
medullary sponge kidney

9. **C D E**
Bartter's syndrome is usually of autosomally recessive inheritance. It classically presents with
   hypokalaemia
   normal blood pressure
   metabolic alkalosis
   vascular insensitivity to pressor agents
   raised plasma renin and aldosterone
   hypertrophy of the juxtaglomerular apparatus.
It has been suggested that it is due to a primary defect in chloride reabsorption in the ascending limb of the loop of Henlé, effectively reducing sodium chloride reabsorption and delivering large amounts to the distal tubule. The Na/K exchange mechanism leads to large losses of potassium. The resultant hypokalaemia triggers prostaglandin release which is behind the vascular insensitivity and defective platelet aggregation.

Clinical signs are growth failure, muscle weakness, constipation and polyuria. Dehydration may occur. Older children can have muscle weakness, cramps and even carpopedal spasm.

Treatment consists of improved nutrition and potassium supplements (with or without sodium). Occasionally indomethacin is required.

10. **ALL FALSE**
There is a high incidence of **urinary tract infection** in children and correct management is essential. Several protocols are recommended; the following is a basic guideline to the management of urinary tract infections in children up to one year of age.
   (i) Ensure there is a definite urinary tract infection ie by a pure growth of 10^5 of an organism (commonly *E. coli*), either by bag sample, clean catch or suprapubic aspiration.
   (ii) Treat the infection with a full course of a sensitve antibiotic, resuscitating and using intravenous medication if warranted.
   (iii) Reculture after full course of antibiotic to ensure infection erradicated and immediately start prophylactic therapy (usually nocturnal trimethoprim).
   (iv) Book an urgent abdominal ultrasound to look for renal abnormalities such as congenital malformation, scarring and hydronephrosis.

Answers and Teaching Notes: Renal Disease

   (v) Arrange a DMSA to assess functional mass of the kidney and a MCUG to assess degree of vesicoureteric reflux. These are usually arranged some three months after the initial urinary tract infection, when the child is clinically well.
  (vi) Ensure the blood pressure has been monitored.
 (vii) Arrange regular follow-up to monitor growth and urine cultures for signs of breakthrough infection.

Grade I vesicoureteric reflux usually completely resolves with appropriate treatment and rarely needs surgical intervention.

11. B C D E

Congenital nephrotic syndrome has an autosomal recessive mode of inheritance. It is more common in Scandinavia than in the United Kingdom, hence the title Finnish type congenital nephrotic syndrome. Light microscopy demonstrates normal glomeruli and cystic dilatation of the proximal tubules. Electron microscopy demonstrates fusion of glomerular basement membrane foot processes.

The neonate may become oedematous, with severe hypoalbuminaemia and highly selective proteinuria.

Antenatally the alpha-fetoprotein is raised, the placenta is abnormally large (25% of birth weight) and the infant is usually premature.

Management tends to be palliative with diuretic, low salt intake and gamma globulin. Death generally occurs from renal failure by two years. More recently trials of bilateral nephrectomy with dialysis and later transplant are being attempted.

12. A C D E

Causes of hypokalaemic metabolic alkalosis include:
    Conn's syndrome
    Cushing's syndrome
    congenital adrenal hyperplasia
    renal artery stenosis
    diuretic abuse.

GASTROENTEROLOGY

1. **Blind loop syndrome**

   - [ ] A occurs in Crohn's disease
   - [ ] B consists of colonisation of the colon with enteric bacteria
   - [ ] C leads to excessive vitamin B12 absorption
   - [ ] D may diminish disaccharidase activity
   - [ ] E may lead to steatorrhoea

2. **Chloride-losing diarrhoea**

   - [ ] A is associated with maternal oligohydramnios
   - [ ] B has onset of symptoms usually after the first 6–8 weeks of life
   - [ ] C is a mild condition
   - [ ] D usually resolves once solids are started
   - [ ] E causes a metabolic alkalosis

3. **Abetalipoproteinaemia**

   - [ ] A is an X-linked inherited condition
   - [ ] B has characteristic erythrocytes
   - [ ] C may present with an ataxic neuropathy
   - [ ] D is associated with retinitis pigmentosa
   - [ ] E consists of defective protein carriage

4. **Electrolyte composition of gastric juice (mmol/l):**

   - [ ] A hydrogen 40-60
   - [ ] B sodium 20-80
   - [ ] C bicarbonate 10-20
   - [ ] D potassium 5-20
   - [ ] E chloride 100-150

5. **Coeliac disease is associated with**

- A iron deficiency anaemia
- B herpes stomatitis
- C HLA B8
- D small bowel malignancy
- E diabetes mellitus

6. **A 13-month-old boy presents with a history of screaming episodes, drawing up his legs and appearing pale. There is a sausage shaped mass in the area of his splenic flexure on palpation.**

- A there is commonly an early history of 'redcurrent jelly'
- B he would be best managed by an air enema study initially
- C conservative treatment such as 'drip and suck' should be considered
- D there may be an increased risk of developing vitamin B12 deficiency in the future if extensive resection is required
- E this condition does not recur

7. **Wilson's disease**

- A is inherited in an autosomal dominant fashion
- B rarely has an onset in childhood
- C if treated by penicillamine should have that drug stopped if proteinuria develops
- D may be kept in remission with zinc salts
- E commonly demonstrates Kayser-Fleischer rings in the early stages of the disease

8. **Blood in the stool of a neonate**

- A if seen on day 1 may be maternal
- B commonly is due to a Meckel's diverticulum
- C may be due to a volvulus
- D may be a presentation of haemorrhagic disease of the newborn
- E is commonly due to Henoch-Schonlein purpura

Gastroenterology

9. Pancreatitis may be caused by

- [ ] A sarcoidosis
- [ ] B systemic lupus erythematosus
- [ ] C choledochal cyst
- [ ] D alpha-1 antitrypsin deficiency
- [ ] E hyperparathyroidism

10. The ascitic fluid in the following conditions is exudative:

- [ ] A congestive heart failure
- [ ] B portal vein obstruction
- [ ] C peritoneal malignancy
- [ ] D cirrhosis
- [ ] E tuberculous peritonitis

11. These symptoms occur more commonly in Crohn's disease than in ulcerative colitis:

- [ ] A hepatic involvement
- [ ] B small bowel malabsorption
- [ ] C perianal disease
- [ ] D mouth ulcers
- [ ] E bloody nocturnal diarrhoea

12. These conditions may cause steatorrhoea:

- [ ] A pancreatic lipase replacement supplements
- [ ] B giardiasis
- [ ] C coeliac disease
- [ ] D abetalipoproteinaemia
- [ ] E Schwachman syndrome

13. Increased mucosal permeability to protein is seen in

- [ ] A primary intestinal lymphangiectasia
- [ ] B graft versus host disease
- [ ] C constrictive pericarditis
- [ ] D Hodgkin's disease
- [ ] E radiation enteritis

14. Hirschsprung's disease

- [ ] A may present with constipation
- [ ] B affects males four times more frequently than females
- [ ] C may present with enterocolitis
- [ ] D characteristically presents with neonatal meconium aspiration syndrome
- [ ] E is associated with delayed passage of barium following enema studies

15. Appendicitis

- [ ] A invariably has a high peripheral white cell count, $30 \times 10^9/1$
- [ ] B can rarely be associated with diarrhoea, tachycardia and flushing
- [ ] C can present with back pain
- [ ] D leading to appendicular abcesses may completely resolve and not require surgical intervention
- [ ] E has lymphoid hyperplasia as an implicated cause

ANSWERS AND TEACHING NOTES : GASTROENTEROLOGY

1. **A D E**
   Blind (or stagnant) loop syndrome occurs when there is stasis of the small intestine contents in the upper regions. This usually occurs when there is incomplete obstruction for example congenitally (malrotation with duodenal bands) or acquired (long standing Crohn's disease). Enteric bacteria are able to colonise the upper small bowel. These bacteria deconjugate bile salts leading to inefficient processing of dietary fat and development of steatorrhoea. Megaloblastic anaemia may occur from interference with vitamin B12 absorption and diarrhoea from disaccharidase deficiency.

2. **E**
   Chloride-losing diarrhoea is a rare specific congenital defect of ileal chloride transport associated with maternal polyhydramnios. The predominant symptom is watery diarrhoea commencing at birth. This occurs secondarily to an increased chloride ion concentration within the intestinal lumen. Later onset can occur but is rare. Dehydration and hypokalaemic, hypochloraemic metabolic alkalosis develop. Infants are often premature and develop hyperbilirubinaemia. Growth and motor development are retarded.

   Management consists of potassium supplements and chloride restriction. The prognosis is variable.

3. **B C D**
   Abetalipoproteinaemia is a rare congenital disease believed to be of autosomal recessive inheritance. It consists of fat malabsorption, acanthocytosis of the red blood cells, ataxic neuropathy and retinitis pigmentosa. There is believed to be an inability to form normal chylomicrons and accordingly defective release and transport of triglycerides from the enterocyte.

   Infants may be normal at birth but develop failure to thrive over the first year. Stools are pale and bulky. Intellectual development is often slightly delayed. After ten years, evidence of ataxic neuropathy develops with loss of deep tendon reflexes and proprioception. By adolescence retinitis pigmentosa can be identified.

   There is no treatment but large supplements of fat soluble vitamins A, D, E and K are given, further massive doses of vitamin E may arrest the neurological degeneration. Reducing the long chain fatty acid intake may alleviate intestinal symptoms.

Answers and Teaching Notes: Gastroenterology

4. **A B D E**
   Electrolyte concentrations in various body compartments (mmol/l)

	Plasma	Intra-Cellular	Gastric Juices
Sodium	140	12	60
Potassium	4	150	9
Chloride	103	4	84
Bicarbonate	25	12	0

5. **A C D E**
   Coeliac disease is associated with small bowel lymphoma.
   Other features include failure to thrive, short stature, abnormally pale faeces, with iron or folate deficiency and vitamin D malabsorption, arising from steatorrhoea. There may be vitamin K deficiency giving rise to hypoprothrombinaemia. Hypoalbuminaemia may also be a feature.
   Dermatitis herpetiformis is associated with coeliac disease and is commonly found on the elbows and other extensor surfaces. The lesions comprise raised papules and vesicles, and are pruritic. These lesions may still remain despite adequate treatment of coeliac disease with a gluten-free diet.
   The average incidence in the UK is 1 in 2000 rising to 1 in 300 in Western Ireland.

6. **B D**
   Intussusception refers to the involution of one part of the bowel into another part, causing obstruction of blood flow to the inner bowel. It is commoner in the first year of life. The ileo-caecal valve is most commonly involved; hence extensive resection may give rise to vitamin B12 deficiency. Children if clinically stable may be managed initially by air enema reduction of the intussusception. Barium enema has lost favour as cases of chemical peritonitis arising from gut perforation secondary to ischaemia of the affected bowel have occurred.
   Conservative treatment is not recommended. If air enema fails to reduce the intussusception, surgical reduction is required. There is a quoted risk of 10% recurrence of this condition. 'Redcurrant jelly' is a classic late sign.

7. **D**
   Wilson's disease is inherited in an autosomal recessive mode, with 50% of cases presenting by the age of 15 years.
   Copper chelation is usually carried out by using penicillamine. Its side-effects include hypersensitivity reactions (rash, fever and lymphadenopathy), lupus-like reactions and proteinuria. The hypersensitivity reaction may be controlled with steroid treatment. The proteinuria is not usually sufficiently severe to cease penicillamine.

Answers and Teaching Notes: Gastroenterology

Zinc salts have been found to help maintain the periods of remission even though copper levels remain high.

Kayser-Fleischer rings are usually seen later in the disease and not commonly in the first decade.

8. **A C D**
   Causes in the neonatal period for blood being seeen in the stool include:
   Ingested maternal blood in the first few days of life
   Necrotizing enterocolitis
   Haemorrhagic disease of the newborn
   Volvulus
   Vascular malformations
   Allergic colitis
   Anal fissure
   The Apt test is used to discriminate maternal from neonatal blood.

9. **A B C D E**
   The following agents/diseases have been implicated in pancreatitis:
   Viral infections – Epstein-Barr, hepatitis A, influenza A, mumps
   Bacterial infections/other – *Mycoplasma pneumoniae*, ascariasis
   Biliary duct obstruction – biliary abnormalities such as choledochal cysts or biliary stones
   Duodenal obstruction – annular pancreas, stricture or compression from tumour such as intestinal lymphoma, enteric cyst, posterior penetrating ulcer, trauma
   Metabolic causes – alpha-1 antitrypsin, hyperlipidaemia
   Systemic illness – Henoch-Schonlein purpura, cystic fibrosis, Crohn's disease, sarcoidosis, hyperparathyroidism, systemic lupus erythematosus

10. **C E**
    Transudative ascitic fluid arises from an increase in hydrostatic pressure in the capillary and lymphatic beds. This produces a clear fluid, with a specific gravity less than 1.015 and protein content less than 2.5 g/dl.

    Conditions which can cause a transudative ascitic fluid collection include:
    Congestive heart failure
    Inferior vena cava obstruction
    Hepatic venous obstruction
    Portal venous thrombosis
    Cirrhosis

Answers and Teaching Notes: Gastroenterology

Exudates are generally turbid, with a specific gravity greater than 1.015 and protein content greater than 2.5 g/dl. Causes include:
Infective peritonitis
Pancreatitis
Peritoneal malignancy.

11. B C D

Bloody nocturnal diarrhoea occurs mostly in ulcerative colitis, whereas weight loss and abdominal pain tend to be the primary symptoms seen in Crohn's disease.

Ulcerative colitis is limited to the mucosa involving the rectum in 95% of cases. It may extend to the level of the ileo-caecal valve and the terminal ileum.

Crohn's disease may involve the whole of the gastro-intestinal tract from mouth to anus. Histologically there is transmural inflammation with non-caseating granulomata.

Ulcerative colitis is associated with an increased incidence of pericholangitis.

Arthritis, uveitis, pyoderma gangrenosum, clubbing, nephrolithiasis and failure to thrive are seen in both conditions.

12. B C D E

Extensive mucosal injury in giardiasis may prevent fat absorption, as in coeliac disease. Allergic gastroenteropathy may have the same pathophysiology.

Defects in lipid transport such as abetalipoproteinaemia, hypobetalipoproteinaemia and chylomicron retention disease can cause steatorrhoea as may lymphangiectasia with lymphatic obstruction.

Pancreatic insufficency is probably the commonest cause, as seen in cystic fibrosis and Schwachman syndrome. However, drugs such as neomycin and cholestyramine also alter bile and bowel flora.

Bile acid deficency eg. biliary atresia or stenosis or intrahepatic cholestasis can also decrease micelle formation.

Absorption may also be disrupted because of extensive ileal dysfunction, eg. caused by surgical removal, Crohn's disease and primary bile salt malabsorption.

13. B E

Protein loss in the bowel may be due either to an increased permeability to plasma/interstitial fluid or to an altered intestinal and mesenteric flow, in which case lymphocytes and chylomicrons are also lost.

Conditions associated with an increased permeability:
Hypertrophic gastritis
Polyposis
Cows' milk allergy

Graft versus host disease
Ulcerative colitis
Enterocolitis
Coeliac disease
Lymphatic abnormality
Primary intestinal lymphangiectasis
Secondary causes: Congestive heart failure
                    Constrictive pericarditis
                    Hodgkin's disease
                    Tuberculosis
                    Lymphoma

Both these pathophysiological mechanisms are seen in radiation enteritis and Crohn's disease.

14. A B C E

Hirschsprung's disease affects 1:5000 live births and may present in the neonatal period with enterocolitis and severe shock. It may also present with abdominal distension, delayed passage of meconium by 24 hours or a complete failure of bowel opening from birth. Chronic constipation may be a feature too. The disease is due to failure of development of ganglion cells, with an increased number of nerve trunks lying in the intermuscular and sub-mucosal areas. The distance affected may vary from an ultra short segment where there is an abnormal sphincter response to a long segment affecting the whole colon.

Barium contrast reveals the transition from normally innervated bowel to a 'cone' shape with a characteristic delay in the passage of barium. Mucosal biopsy is mandatory to assess the level and extent of involvement.

Surgical treatment is a mainstay of treatment depending on the length of the affected bowel.

15. B C E

Appendicitis can occur at any age, with obstruction giving rise to the increase in the pressure of the intraluminal wall causing haemorrhage, thrombosis, oedema and secondary bacterial infection.

Lymphoid hyperplasia, adhesions and faecoliths can cause obstruction. Inflammation of the appendix then leads to necrosis and perforation. Signs of peritonism may be obscured by the omentum sealing around it.

Carcinoid may be a cause, giving tachycardia, diarrhoea and flushing. Back pain may represent a retrocaecal position and appendicular masses require surgery as cases of recurrence have been described.

METABOLIC DISORDERS

1. **Classic phenylketonuria**

   - [ ] A is caused by deficiency of phenylalanine
   - [ ] B requires total exclusion of phenylalanine from the diet
   - [ ] C results in mild mental retardation if untreated
   - [ ] D may be affected by the development of a seborrhoeic rash
   - [ ] E in infancy is typified by hypertonicity

2. **Classic homocystinuria**

   - [ ] A is a defect in metabolism of tyrosine
   - [ ] B is inherited as an autosomal recessive trait
   - [ ] C responds to high doses of vitamin B6 in 40% of cases
   - [ ] D is usually diagnosed soon after birth
   - [ ] E may be confused with Marfan's syndrome

3. **Hartnup disease**

   - [ ] A leads to grossly elevated plasma amino acid levels
   - [ ] B is associated with aminoaciduria
   - [ ] C is associated with low plasma tryptophan levels
   - [ ] D leads to skin photosensitivity
   - [ ] E is associated with cerebellar ataxia

4. **Biotin deficiency**

   - [ ] A is typified by presentation soon after birth
   - [ ] B is associated with episodes of metabolic alkalosis
   - [ ] C is not a treatable condition
   - [ ] D may present with ataxia
   - [ ] E is frequently associated with dementia

Metabolic Disorders

5. Nonketotic hyperglycinaemia

- [ ] A carries an excellent prognosis
- [ ] B is suggested by mothers noticing hiccoughs in utero
- [ ] C is associated with myoclonic type seizures
- [ ] D usually presents after the first few months of life
- [ ] E may be diagnosed antenatally

6. Ornithine transcarbamylase deficiency

- [ ] A does not occur in females
- [ ] B is an X-linked dominant condition
- [ ] C is always diagnosed in the first month of life
- [ ] D can be diagnosed by prenatal fetal liver biopsy
- [ ] E produces a Reye-like syndrome

7. Type IIa glycogen storage disease

- [ ] A has classic ECG changes
- [ ] B is due to an acid maltase deficiency
- [ ] C may be confused with Werdnig-Hoffman disease on presentation
- [ ] D is also called McArdle's disease
- [ ] E may present in infancy with severe paralysis and hypotonia

8. In the mucopolysaccharidoses

- [ ] A the commonest form is Hunter's
- [ ] B Hurler's is of X-linked inheritance
- [ ] C children with Hunter's have cataracts
- [ ] D the Sanfillipo form is associated with profound mental retardation
- [ ] E the Morquio form is associated with severe bony changes

9. Calcium

- [ ] A bound to plasma proteins accounts for 4% of the total plasma concentration
- [ ] B is physiologically active only in the ionised form
- [ ] C has a normal ionised range of 2–2.5 mmol/l
- [ ] D in the ionised form accounts for 50% of the total blood calcium
- [ ] E may be reduced following cardio-pulmonary bypass

10. Potassium

- [ ] A daily requirements are about 10–20 mmol/kg/day
- [ ] B in serum concentration at 9 mmol produces peaked P waves
- [ ] C serum concentration increases following administration of insulin
- [ ] D is predominantly an extracellular anion
- [ ] E is directly maintained in electrolyte balance by vasopressin

ANSWERS AND TEACHING NOTES : METABOLIC DISORDERS

1. **D E**
   This autosomal recessive condition develops secondary to deficiency of phenylalanine hydroxylase, leading to failure of conversion of phenylalanine to tyrosine. Consequent build up of phenylalanine results in progressive mental retardation with hypertonicity and brisk deep reflexes in sleeping infants. Chidren often have fair hair and blue eyes, further they may develop a seborrhoeic or eczematous rash. Vomiting can be a severe problem. Children develop hyperactivity and purposeless movements, rhythmic rocking and athetosis. They may have an unusual odour described as musty or mousey. About a quarter of cases have fitting. Clinically there is microcephaly, prominent maxilla with widely spaced teeth, enamel hypoplasia and growth retardation. Management is essentially via the diet consisting of partial but not total exclusion of phenylalanine as it remains an essential amino acid.

2. **B C E**
   Homocystinaemia type I or classic homocystinuria is a result of a defect in metabolism of methionine, it is inherited by the autosomal recessive route and about 40% of cases will respond to high dose vitamin B6. Diagnosis tends to be after 3 years of age with eye changes (eg. subluxation of the lens, glaucoma, cataracts and optic atrophy). There may be developmental delay and failure to thrive evident in retrospect. Mental retardation is generally progressive without intervention and fitting occurs in about 3% of cases. Clinical features resemble Marfan's syndrome with the tall thin stature, arachnodactyly and high arched palate.

3. **B C D E**
   Hartnup disease is a very rare disorder caused by a defect in the transport of monoamino-monocarboxylic amino acids by the renal tubules and intestinal mucosa. Plasma amino acid levels are normal except for tryptophan which secondary to excess renal tubular loss and impaired intestinal uptake is low. Massive generalised aminoaciduria occurs. Clinical features include severe skin rashes on exposure to sunlight and development of cerebellar ataxia. Mental retardation is not a recognised complication.

4. **D E**
   Biotin deficiency occurs secondary to a defect in biotinidase production. It usually presents from a few months to even a few years of age. Symptoms include dementia, ataxia, seizures, hair loss and immunodeficiency. Episodes of metabolic acidosis may occur. Children are treated with biotin, usually with a very good response.

Answers and Teaching Notes: Metabolic Disorders

5. **B C E**
   This serious condition usually presents in the first few days of life with poor feeding, lethargy and gradual onset of coma. Infants have myoclonic seizures and mothers may comment on having noticed in utero hiccoughs. The condition carries a very poor prognosis with no effective treatment. It is believed to be autosomally recessively inherited and can now be diagnosed by antenatal analysis of glycine and serine levels in amniotic fluid.

6. **D E**
   This X-linked recessive condition severely affects males and affects females to a far lesser extent. Male infants present in the first few days of life with hyperammonaemia and are generally extremely unwell. They occasionally present in a Reye syndrome type state. Infants may present as cot-deaths. Affected females can give a history of intermittent encephalopathic episodes, exacerbated by protein loads. Perinatal diagnosis is now possible by fetal liver biopsy.

7. **A B C E**
   Type IIa glycogenosis (or Pompes disease in infantile presentation) is due to a deficiency of acid maltase. There is multisystem involvement of skeletal muscle, heart, liver, CNS and kidneys. Presentation in infancy is with severe paralysis and hypotonia, also cardiac or respiratory compromise may occur. There may be confusion with Werdig-Hoffman disease. The prognosis is very poor.

   Diagnosis may be suggested by ECG findings of short PR interval, depressed ST segments and inverted T waves. Peripheral blood film shows deposition of glycogen in the lymphocytes. Assay of acid maltase in cultured fibroblasts allows prenatal diagnosis by chorionic villus sampling and is the investigation of choice postnatally. Muscle biopsy shows severely distorted fibres with massive glycogen deposition and strong acid phosphatase activity.

8. **D E**
   The commonest type of **mucopolysaccharidosis** is the Sanfillipo form. All forms are believed to be of autosomal recessive inheritance except Hunter's which is X-linked.

	Bony changes	Large liver/spleen	*Mental retardation*	*Corneal clouding*
Hurler's	+	+	+	+
Hunter's	+	+	+	−
Sanfillipo	+/−	+/−	+	−
Morquio	+++	−	−	+
Maroteaux Lamy	+++	+	−	+

Answers and Teaching Notes: Metabolic Disorders

9. **B D E**
   45% of total plasma calcium exists bound to plasma proteins such as albumin, 5% is complexed in the plasma (eg. as citrated forms) and the remainder (50%) is in the ionised form. This ionised form is the physiologically active form and may be reduced following cardiopulmonary bypass. The normal range for ionised calcium is 1.05–1.25 mmol/l.

10. **ALL FALSE**
    Daily potassium requirements are about 1–2 mmol/kg/day. Potassium is a predominantly intracellular cation with a normal serum range of 3.5–5 mmol/l.

    Insulin in combination with dextrose is used in the treatment of hyperkalaemia, causing increased cellular uptake.

    Abnormal ECG changes include tented T waves, followed by widened QRS complexes and cardiac arrest.

ENDOCRINOLOGY

1. **Septo-optic dysplasia**

   - [ ] A consists of bilateral optic nerve hypoplasia and the absence of the septum pellucidum
   - [ ] B is a benign condition
   - [ ] C usually consists of defects in thyroid function
   - [ ] D may present in the neonatal period with prolonged jaundice
   - [ ] E is associated with hypoglycaemia secondary to hyperinsulinism

2. **McCune-Albright syndrome**

   - [ ] A may be confused with neurofibromatosis
   - [ ] B is associated with thyroid dysfunction
   - [ ] C has an increased incidence of Addison's disease
   - [ ] D is more common in boys
   - [ ] E is characterised by the development of precocious puberty by 3 years

3. **Pseudohypoparathyroidism**

   - [ ] A consists of raised PTH levels in the presence of hypercalcaemia
   - [ ] B is associated with above average intelligence
   - [ ] C is associated with short stature
   - [ ] D has an increased incidence of cataracts
   - [ ] E is associated most commonly with shortening of the 2nd metacarpal of the index finger

4. **Causes of hypercalcaemia without PTH excess include**

   - [ ] A hypothyroidism
   - [ ] B vitamin A deficiency
   - [ ] C tuberculosis
   - [ ] D Williams' syndrome
   - [ ] E post kidney transplantation

Endocrinology

5. The following endocrine disorders can be detected by cDNA probes:

- [ ] A McCune-Albright syndrome
- [ ] B testicular feminisation syndrome
- [ ] C Laron dwarfism
- [ ] D vitamin D resistant rickets
- [ ] E pseudohypoparathyroidism

6. Addison's disease

- [ ] A in the last century was primarily due to tuberculosis
- [ ] B is usually due to autoimmune disease
- [ ] C is often due to amyloidosis in children
- [ ] D may be associated with chronic mucocutaneous candidiasis
- [ ] E presents with acute hypokalaemic, hypotensive crises

7. Pseudohermaphroditism is associated with

- [ ] A Wilms' tumour
- [ ] B neuroblastoma
- [ ] C end stage renal failure
- [ ] D cataracts
- [ ] E sporadic aniridia

8. Growth charts

- [ ] A exist specifically for patients with achondroplasia
- [ ] B specifically for children with Down's syndrome are available
- [ ] C can be accurately used to diagnose hydrocephalus on first presentation
- [ ] D produce a wide range of variability in readings
- [ ] E cannot be used to compare with parental size

Endocrinology

9. Synacthen tests

- [ ] A may be used to identify an enzyme deficiency
- [ ] B causing a 2–3 fold increase in cortisol would be abnormal
- [ ] C require children to be fasted beforehand
- [ ] D require children to be monitored throughout with regular blood glucose tests
- [ ] E of short type should be used to rule out secondary adrenal insufficiency

10. The following changes occur in:

- [ ] A pseudohypoparathyroidism = low Ca, high PO_4 and low PTH
- [ ] B rickets (of vitamin D deficiency) = high Ca, low PO_4, high alkaline phosphatase and normal/high PTH
- [ ] C vitamin D resistant rickets = low PTH and high PO_4
- [ ] D hypoparathyroidism = low Ca, low PO_4 and very low PTH
- [ ] E vitamin D dependent rickets = low PTH

11. The water deprivation test

- [ ] A assesses aldosterone production
- [ ] B is a safe investigation
- [ ] C should be performed in infants after at least a 16 hour fast
- [ ] D must have accurate starting weights recorded
- [ ] E can be used to pick up X-linked carriers of diabetes insipidus

12. Raised growth hormone levels without excessive stature may occur with

- [ ] A malnutrition
- [ ] B Silver-Russell syndrome
- [ ] C poorly controlled diabetes
- [ ] D craniopharyngioma
- [ ] E Laron syndrome

Endocrinology

13. A 2-year-old child is found to have a destructive lesion of the hypothalamus. She is likely to have

- [ ] A excessive anterior pituitary hormone release
- [ ] B disturbed water balance
- [ ] C weight loss
- [ ] D a glioma
- [ ] E temperature instability

14. A 2-day-old baby is transferred to SCBU following poor feeding on the postnatal ward. The baby appears hypovolaemic and on close examination the genitalia are ambiguous. It is necessary to

- [ ] A consider congenital adrenal hyperplasia secondary to 11-OH deficiency
- [ ] B measure plasma 17 alpha-OH progesterone levels at day 3
- [ ] C reassure parents of child's correct sex
- [ ] D commence replacement therapy
- [ ] E arrange genetic counselling

15. Increased thyroid binding globulin levels are found in

- [ ] A pregnancy
- [ ] B nephrotic syndrome
- [ ] C acute hepatitis
- [ ] D androgen therapy
- [ ] E cirrhosis

ANSWERS AND TEACHING NOTES : ENDOCRINOLOGY

1. **A D**
   Septo-optic dysplasia is refered to as bilateral optic nerve hypoplasia in the absence of the septum pellucidum. It can be an extremely serious condition if not detected early as the degree of hypothalamic involvement varies widely. The commonest finding is of growth hormone deficiency alone but multiple abnormalities may occur including disastrous effects from diabetes insipidus. Newborn infants may present with hypotonia, apnoea, prolonged jaundice, seizures and hypoglycaemia without hyperinsulinism. Males are associated with the finding of micropenis. The condition is believed to be sporadic but increased incidence does occur with consanguinity.

2. **A B E**
   McCune-Albright syndrome is characterised by polyostotic fibrous dysplasia of the skeletal system, irregular edged cafe-au-lait spots and endocrine dysfunction, namely precocious puberty but also hyperthyroidism and Cushing's syndrome. It is far more common in girls than in boys. The average age for menarche in girls is around 3 years, although symtoms are occasionally noticed far earlier.
   Since neurofibromatosis also presents with cutaneous lesions (usually smooth outlined cafe-au-lait spots), increased incidence of precocious puberty and bony abnormalities, confusion can occasionally arise.

3. **C D**
   Pseudohypoparathyroidism is a condition due to a genetic defect in the receptor tissues. Accordingly there are normal or raised parathyroid hormone levels but continuing hypocalcaemia. There is a wide range of clinical manifestations but classically individuals are of short stature, with mental retardation, lenticular cataracts and shortening of the 2nd metacarpal and metatarsal of the fourth and fifth digits. Calcification of the basal ganglia is found. Children may present with tetany.

4. **C D**
   Causes of hypercalcaemia without PTH excess:
   Williams' syndrome
   tuberculosis
   sarcoidosis
   malignancy e.g. leukaemia, lymphoma, neuroblastoma, bone tumours
   prolonged immobility
   hypervitaminosis A
   vitamin D excess
   hyperthyroidism
   subcutaneous fat necrosis
   Addison's disease

Answers and Teaching Notes: Endocrinology

Causes of hypercalcaemia with hyperparathyroidism:
Primary hyperparathyroidism
Secondary hyperparathyroidism eg. post renal transplant
Transient neonatal hyperparathyroidism with maternal hypoparathyroidism.

5. **B C D**
Present conditions detectable by cDNA probes are:
Laron dwarfism
Testicular feminisation syndrome
Vitamin D resistant rickets
Congenital adrenal hyperplasia (especially 21-hydroxylase deficiency)
Familial ADH deficiency
Multiple endocrine neoplasia syndrome
Prader-Willi syndrome

6. **A B D**
Addison's disease was previously mainly found in association with tuberculous involvement of the adrenal gland. Present day cases are most commonly of autoimmune disease. Amyloid is an adult cause of the disorder.

Addison's is involved in type I and II autoimmune polyglandular syndrome.

Type I	Addison's disease
	hypoparathyroidism
	chronic mucocutaneous candidiasis
	increased incidence of alopecia, malabsorption, pernicious anaemia, gonadal failure, chronic active hepatitis and vitiligo.
	There is no HLA association.
Type II	Addison's disease
	autoimmune thyroid disease
	insulin-dependent diabetes
	predominance of HLA DR3 and HLA DR4.

Presentation may be with gradual weight loss, increased skin pigmentation and muscle weakness, but acute crises occur with severe hypotension, hypoglycaemia, hyponatraemia and hyperkalaemia which constitutes a medical emergency.

7. **A C E**
There are two **syndromes linked with pseudohermaphroditism**:

Answers and Teaching Notes: Endocrinology

(i) DRASH – Wilms' tumour
glomerulonephropathy leading to end stage renal failure
pseudohermaphroditism
(ii) WAGER – Wilms' tumour
pseudohermaphroditism
mental retardation
sporadic aniridia

This is associated with deletions on the short arm of chromosome 11.

8. **A B D**
Growth charts are vital to monitoring the child's general development. Special charts for specific conditions exist notably Down's syndrome, achondroplasia and Turner's syndrome. The aim of growth charts is to provide a spread of values over a period of time monitoring the trend in height, weight and head circumference and thus growth velocity. Accordingly a single value for head circumference would be impossible to interpret even if it was above the 97th centile. The child's other centile plottings must be noted to see if they too are above the 97th centile and the trend in head circumference growth looked into to ensure no rapid expansion has occurred. Further it is essential to plot the parents' details on the far side of the chart to compare them with their child's. Unfortunately great observer error is inevitable with these recordings, for example only occasionally weighing the child undressed, weighing babies immediately after a feed and of course variation between scales. Similar problems with height recordings can also occur.

9. **A**
An ACTH stimulation or synacthen test is used to demonstrate adrenal insufficiency or to identify an enzyme deficiency by triggering an increase in the precursor steroid production. For short and prolonged tests fasting is not required and children should not have problems with drops in their blood sugar levels. The short test takes just over an hour. The prolonged test consists of priming for 3 days with synacthen depot (tetracosactrin acetate) intramuscular injections before sampling cortisol levels. A 2–3 fold increase in cortisol in the short test and a 3 fold increase in the prolonged test would be expected in normal subjects. A poor response would suggest primary or secondary adrenal insufficiency, whilst no cortisol response after the prolonged test would confirm primary adrenal insufficiency. The prolonged synacthen test should usually result in a cortisol response in secondary adrenal insufficiency where a remnant of previously understimulated adrenal tissue remains.

Answers and Teaching Notes: Endocrinology

10. **ALL FALSE**

	Ca	PO$_4$	ALP	PTH
Hypoparathyroidism	low	high	N	low/zero
Pseudohypoparathyroidism	low	high	N/high	high
Rickets (vit. D deficiency)	N/low	low	high	high
Vit. D resistant rickets	N/low	very low	high	N
Vit. D dependent rickets	N/low	low	high	N/high

11. **D E**

    Water deprivation test is carried out in situations where diabetes insipidus is suspected. It is essential to have an accurate starting weight, initial blood sodium, osmolality and ADH (if available) and urine osmolality. Children usually do not require fasting for more than 12–16 hours to establish an answer and in infants it can be extremely dangerous to fast for more than 8 hours, especially in genuine cases of diabetes insipidus. Blood and urine samples are taken at regular intervals and in situations of excessive urinary losses with no apparent concentration, intranasal or intramuscular DDAVP may be given. Consequent concentration of urine may then be seen in deficient states. Cases that continue to loose dilute urine and are shown to have raised ADH levels are often found to be nephrogenic diabetes insipidus. Similarly carriers of this X-linked disorder can be picked up by their slightly reduced responsivenes to ADH, even with raised levels.

12. **A C E**

    Malnutrition, poorly controlled diabetes and growth hormone resistance all lead to raised growth hormone levels without excessive growth. In Laron syndrome large amounts of active growth hormone are secreted, but fail to generate somatomedin C, so growth does not occur.

    Silver-Russell syndrome is characterised by short stature, frontal bossing, small triangular facies, sparse subcutaneous tissue and shortened, incurved fifth fingers. Growth hormone levels are usually normal.

13. **B D E**

    Destructive lesions of the hypothalamus cause deficiences in releasing hormones, disturb water balance (due to diabetes insipidus), and give rise to temperature instability. The child is more likely to have hyperphagia and obesity than weight loss. The destructive lesion may be to a glioma, dysgerminoma or craniopharyngioma.

14. **B D E**

    This baby is more likely to have congenital adrenal hyperplasia secondary to 21 alpha hydroxylase deficiency than 11 hydroxylase deficiency, as the blood pressure drops and hypovolaemia occurs in the former; 11 hydroxylase deficiency tends to present after the neonatal period with raised blood pressure and hypokalaemia. It is important

Answers and Teaching Notes: Endocrinology

to measure the plasma 17 alpha-OH progesterone levels at day 3 as these are raised in salt losing states whereas normal babies tend to have high levels on the first and second day of life which then drop. The levels are persistently raised in congenital adrenal hyperplasia.

It is unwise to tell parents the sex of the child until treatment is started and controlled, as the phenotypic appearance may change.

Replacement therapy is essential for survival, using mineralocorticoid and hydrocortisone.

Genetic counselling is indicated as this condition is transmitted by autosomal recessive inheritance. The gene is located on the short arm of chromosome 6.

Ninety-five percent of cases are due to 21 alpha hydroxylase deficiency.

Prenatal diagnosis is possible as raised levels of 17 OH progesterone and androstenedione are found in the amniotic fluid.

HLA typing of fetus and affected siblings permits confirmation of diagnosis and the detection of heterozygotes.

An adrenocortical tumour may cause virilization and should be considered as a differential diagnosis.

15. **A C**
   Increased thyroid binding globulins are found in:
   oestrogen
   contraceptive and clofibrate therapy
   pregnancy
   the newborn period
   acute hepatitis
   narcotic abuse
   congenital excess (X-linked dominant)

   Decreased thyroid binding globulins are found in:
   congenital deficiency (X-linked dominant)
   nephrotic syndrome
   severe liver failure
   anabolic steroids
   androgens
   glucocorticoids
   L-asparaginase in cytotoxic therapy

   Abnormalities of thyroid binding globulin are not necessarily of clinical importance, but they may lead to misdiagnosis of hypo- or hyperthyroidism.

NEUROLOGY

1. **Gilles de la Tourette syndrome**

   - [ ] A occurs only in boys
   - [ ] B does not occur below 8 years of age
   - [ ] C responds well to treatment
   - [ ] D is rarer in Japan than in the United Kingdom
   - [ ] E does not demonstrate twitches during sleep

2. **Duchenne muscular dystrophy**

   - [ ] A has equal sex incidence
   - [ ] B is associated with language delay
   - [ ] C presents with distal lower limb weakness
   - [ ] D is associated with a negative Gower's sign
   - [ ] E classically has brisk knee and ankle reflexes with upgoing plantars

3. **Diagnosis of Duchenne muscular dystrophy**

   - [ ] A cannot be carried by DNA analysis
   - [ ] B is confirmed by raised ESR
   - [ ] C is reinforced by raised CPK
   - [ ] D is accompanied by frequent ECG findings
   - [ ] E is often confirmed on muscle biopsy

4. **The congenital form of dystrophia myotonica**

   - [ ] A is associated with major neonatal feeding problems
   - [ ] B is complicated by severe epilepsy
   - [ ] C usually presents with cataracts and frontal balding
   - [ ] D classically presents with neonatal hypertonicity
   - [ ] E is associated with universally severe mental retardation

5. Mitochondrial cytopathy is associated with

- [ ] A retinitis pigmentosa
- [ ] B autosomal recessive inheritance
- [ ] C short stature
- [ ] D ataxia
- [ ] E diagnosis on muscle biopsy

6. Kernicterus induced cerebral palsy

- [ ] A is frequently related to damage to the basal ganglia
- [ ] B is associated with athetoid movements
- [ ] C is associated with severe mental retardation
- [ ] D can cause a defect of upward gaze
- [ ] E has an increased incidence of deafness

7. Ataxia telangiectasia

- [ ] A is an autosomal dominant condition
- [ ] B usually presents with cerebellar ataxia
- [ ] C typically has the classic skin lesions clearly visible by three years
- [ ] D is associated with fitting in the majority of cases
- [ ] E does not affect intelligence

8. Ataxia telangiectasia is associated with

- [ ] A nasal sinusitis and middle ear disease
- [ ] B tonsillar hypertrophy
- [ ] C defective immunoglobulin synthesis
- [ ] D development of leukaemia
- [ ] E glucose intolerance

9. Dandy-Walker syndrome

- [ ] A classically presents with dilated third and lateral ventricles
- [ ] B often clinically demonstrates a cerebellar ataxia
- [ ] C should not be shunted
- [ ] D is not associated with mental retardation
- [ ] E may be associated with an occipital encephalocele

10. Moyamoya disease

- [ ] A has a wide range of symptoms on presentation
- [ ] B tends to resolve spontaneously
- [ ] C may result in an acute hemiplegia
- [ ] D is associated with neurofibromatosis
- [ ] E can be safely and non-invasively investigated by hyperventilation during EEG monitoring

11. In Moebius syndrome

- [ ] A there is an absence or maldevelopment of cranial nerve nuclei and their nerves
- [ ] B the fifth cranial nerve is most often affected
- [ ] C birth trauma may lead to the condition
- [ ] D the face may be expressionless
- [ ] E there is an association with mental deficiency

12. The Dubowitz score

- [ ] A estimates gestational age to within three days
- [ ] B is best carried out between weeks 1 and 2 after birth
- [ ] C the better the tone the older gestationally the neonate
- [ ] D the greater the joint laxity the greater the gestational age
- [ ] E uses plantar creases in the scoring system

Neurology

13. The following is true about reflexes present in the normal neonate:

☐ A palmar grasp starts to appear from 34 weeks' gestation
☐ B brisk deep tendon reflexes are present from birth
☐ C more than 10 beats of clonus is abnormal
☐ D an extensor plantar reflex is abnormal
☐ E rooting reflexes occur after 28 weeks' gestation

14. Rolandic epilepsy

☐ A occurs exclusively below 2 years of age
☐ B is a life-long condition
☐ C can occur during sleep
☐ D is associated with learning difficulties
☐ E has classical CT changes

15. Rett syndrome

☐ A is twice as common in girls as in boys
☐ B affects children between 4 to 6 years of age
☐ C is associated with high ammonia levels
☐ D does not affect intelligence
☐ E is characterised by hand wringing

16. A 9-month-old infant is found to have abnormally widened fontanelles. It is important to consider

☐ A rickets
☐ B Alagille's syndrome
☐ C hypothyroidism
☐ D cranio-synostosis
☐ E Rubenstein-Tabyi syndrome

Neurology

17. Acute ataxia may be caused by

- [ ] A alcohol ingestion
- [ ] B hypoglycaemia
- [ ] C cerebellar astrocytoma
- [ ] D neuroblastoma
- [ ] E phenytoin

18. Lennox-Gastaut syndrome

- [ ] A carries a poor prognosis when associated with West's syndrome
- [ ] B consists of more than one type of epilepsy
- [ ] C is usually associated with a normal intelligence quotient
- [ ] D responds to monotherapy
- [ ] E usually regresses in adolescence

19. The following statements are true:

- [ ] A homonymous hemianopia implies a lesion posterior to the optic chiasma
- [ ] B the optic radiation fans out from the lateral geniculate body
- [ ] C pupillary responses are altered if there is third nerve damage
- [ ] D concentric tunnel-like blindness may be seen in hysterical blindness
- [ ] E unilateral blindness may be due to an optic glioma

20. Absent or decreased reflexes may be seen in

- [ ] A Refsum's disease
- [ ] B Riley-Day syndrome
- [ ] C hypothyroidism
- [ ] D spinal muscular atrophy
- [ ] E Guillain-Barré syndrome

21. When considering febrile convulsions:

- ☐ A the incidence of febrile convulsions in infancy is 0.01%
- ☐ B the age of greatest susceptibility is between 1 and 6 months of age
- ☐ C a focus of infection is not required as long as the temperature is above 40 degrees Centigrade
- ☐ D the longer a convulsion lasts the less likely is the risk of recurrence
- ☐ E recurrence rates are of the order of 0.3%

22. Macrocephaly is found in

- ☐ A Edward's syndrome
- ☐ B Tay-Sach's syndrome
- ☐ C achondroplasia
- ☐ D Cornelia de Lange syndrome
- ☐ E neurofibromatosis

ANSWERS AND TEACHING NOTES : NEUROLOGY

1. **E**

   Gilles de la Tourette syndrome consists of compulsive verbal obscenities and recurrent, involuntary, repetitive motor movements. There is the ability to suppress the movements voluntarily for minutes to hours and variation in intensity.

   Age of onset may be between 2–15 years with an average of 7 years. The syndrome is three times more common in boys than in girls. The signs disappear during sleep and become worse with anxiety. The condition is more common in Japan and the USA and rare in the United Kingdom. It responds poorly to treatment, but some cases benefit from haloperidol.

2. **B**

   Duchenne muscular dystrophy is an X-linked recessive condition affecting the proximal lower limbs primarily. It is well known for the classical presentation of Gower's sign, with which the patient gets up from the floor by climbing up his legs.

   Boys usually present by three years with delayed walking or abnormal gait. They frequently have a history of always being thought to have had an abnormal gait by their families. Further intellectual delay is common, especially speech delay.

   Clinically children have marked calf hypertrophy, initially due to overcompensation and later pseudohypertrophy with fatty and connective tissue replacement of muscle tissue. There is a marked lumbar lordosis. Knee jerks are lost early, ankle reflexes often remaining and plantars are usually flexor. There is marked wasting of quadriceps and other proximal lower limb muscles. Weakness and reduced reflexes of the upper limb muscles can occasionally be detected early. Boys are usually wheelchair bound by their early teens and death occurs by 20–25 years. The last stages are frequently intolerable with progressive loss of respiratory function, speech and swallowing, accompanied by contractures and deformities occurring with muscle wastage and immobility.

3. **C D E**

   Duchenne muscular dystrophy can now be detected by an $Xp2$ deletion on DNA analysis for the dystrophin gene. Accordingly carrier females can be picked up. Other relevant investigations include:
   - CPK (which is usually greater than 10 000)
   - EMG (showing myopathic changes)
   - Muscle biopsy (showing increased fatty and connective tissue change, muscle bundle variation in diameter with necrosis and regeneration, evidence of histiocytic infiltration and the tissue will stain poorly for dystrophin).

   Most cases have cardiac involvement. The heart develops extensive patchy fibrosis and disorganised muscle fibres. Death may occur secondary to sudden myocardial failure due to arrhythmias and cardiomyopathy.

4. **A**
Congenital presentation of dystrophia myotonica is usually with severe hypotonia in the neonatal period. Infants are very difficult to feed. They have expressionless faces and open triangular mouths. The initial impression is one of mental retardation but intelligence is often normal. Epilepsy is not a major feature and cataracts and frontal balding are later features of the acquired form. Infants may suffer from apnoeas and episodes of cyanosis secondary to poor respiratory function, diaphragms are often high and there may be a history of early death of previous siblings. A high incidence of polyhydramnios occurs secondary to poor fetal swallowing of amniotic fluid. There is increased incidence of congenital talipes and other joint deformites.

5. **A C D E**
Mitochondrial cytopathy is an abnormality of mitochondria and lipid. Muscle biopsy demonstrates ragged red fibres on staining. Inheritance is non-Mendelian through the mother. Depending on the amount of mitochondrial DNA transmitted, the extent of abnormality can vary markedly from child to child.

A progressive external ophthalmoplegia in association with short stature, ptosis, retinitis pigmentosa, ataxia, sensorineural deafness, mental retardation and limb muscle weakness occurs. Further complications include an autonomic neuropathy and abnormal cardiac conduction often requiring a pacemaker.

6. **A B D E**
Kernicterus induced cerebral palsy is usually associated with a dyskinetic or athetoid form, with purposeless, involuntary movements. There is high-tone hearing loss but intelligence is generally normal. The basal ganglia are often stained with bilirubin and damaged and the dental enamel stained green, with poorly formed teeth. Children are very thin and lacking subcutaneous fat tissue. There is a defect of upward gaze (unlike the post-anoxic cases of dyskinetic cerebral palsy).

7. **B**
Ataxia telangiectasia is of autosomal recessive inheritance. Presentation is usually shortly after the child starts walking when cerebellar ataxia becomes apparent. The lower limbs are initially affected and involvement of the upper limbs comes later, occasionally with titubation and dysarthria. Mental retardation and progressive dementia can occur. Further there is growth retardation and an increased incidence of chest infections.

This progressive disorder usually results in the child being wheelchair bound by 10–12 years and death occurs before adult life from respiratory failure.

The telangiectasia are usually first visible in the conjunctiva after three years of age and become more extensive over the years.

8. **A C D E**
Ataxia telangiectasia is associated with increased incidence of middle ear disease and nasal sinusitis. There is absent or reduced tonsillar tissue and frequently absent thymus. IgA is nearly always reduced, IgG is quite often decreased and IgM has abnormal function. There is increased incidence of lymphoma, sarcoma, leukaemia, Hodgkin's disease, cerebellar neoplasms, ovarian dysgerminomas and gastric cancer. Malignancies are more common in relatives.

Abnormal carbohydrate metabolism is a common finding, in the most extreme form resulting in glucose intolerance with raised insulin levels, and a failure of insulin to reduce blood sugar levels. On investigation alpha-fetoprotein is often found to be raised and cultured lymphocytes and fibroblasts have abnormal sensitivity following irradiation.

9. **B E**
Dandy-Walker syndrome results from an occlusion of the foramina of Lusckha and Magendie of the fourth ventricle. The result is a small, hypoplastic cerebellum and a dilated fourth ventricle, with an enlarged posterior fossa. There may be an associated occipital encephalocele.

Obstructive hydrocephalus and cerebellar ataxia are often features of presentation. Mental retardation which can be severe occurs in about 70% of cases. Shunts are often required not only to the lateral ventricles but also to the cystic fourth ventricle itself.

10. **A C D**
Moyamoya disease or progressive cerebral arterial occlusive disease presents with a wide range of severity and clinical signs. Common presentations include acute hemiplegia, transient dysphasia and other deficits with or without fitting. There is an association with neurofibromatosis.

Hyperventilating is extremely dangerous and markedly increases the risk of fitting, development of neurological signs and having an intracranial bleed.

11. **A D**
Moebius syndrome, also known as congenital nuclear aplasia, consists of absence or maldevelopment of cranial nuclei and their nerves. The facial nerve is most often affected. In the severest form of the syndrome

Answers and Teaching Notes: Neurology

the face may be completely expressionless with facial immobility, difficulty in chewing, swallowing, ptosis and complete ophthalmoplegia.

Other anomalies may occur such as absence of pectoralis muscles and club foot deformities.

The children are not mentally deficient but may have learning difficulties arising from the cranial nerve defects.

12. C E

The Dubowitz score is used to estimate gestational age to within two weeks. It is best carried out on the first day of life, after the neonate has stabilised. As gestational age increases so the tone and limb flexion become greater and joints become less lax. Important features in this scoring system include: oedema, skin texture, skin colour, lanugo, plantar creases, nipple formation, pinna development and genital appearance.

13. B

In the newborn period, the Moro reflex should be present from birth and not disappear until the infant is four to five months old. It is the reflex flexion of limbs particularly of the upper limbs on allowing the head of the infant to drop backwards whilst supporting the spine.

Stepping and placing reflexes are found at birth in term infants.

The palmar grasp is present from 28 weeks onwards. Deep tendon reflexes tend to be brisk initially.

Upto 10 to 20 beats of clonus are normal.

The Babinski reflex is usually extensor in infancy.

Rooting reflex (turning the head to light tactile stimulation in the perioral area) is usually present from 32 weeks.

14. C

Benign focal epilepsy or Rolandic epilepsy tends to occur between 5 and 10 years of age and is rare before 2 years. It accounts for up to 16% of all afebrile seizures below 15 years. Seizures are focal motor with generalised tonic-clonic spread. Over half the children affected have episodes only during sleep or on awakening.

In the awake state, motor or sensory symptoms may occur involving tongue, mouth and face. Speech and swallowing are commonly impaired and the child may be able to understand what is being said to him but be unable to communicate.

A family history is noted in 13% of patients.

Rolandic epilepsy disappears by adolescence or early adulthood. Intelligence is normal and no abnormalities are found on CT scanning.

15. E

Rett syndrome is a neurodegenerative disorder affecting only females with onset at about 1 year of age.

There is loss of purposeful hand movement and communication skills, social withdrawal, gait apraxia, stereotypic repetitive hand movements that resemble hand washing, wringing or clapping of hands and acquired microcephaly.

The condition plateaus for many years before seizures, spasticity and kyphoscoliosis develop.

Metabolic investigations are normal as Rett syndrome is of unknown aetiology.

16. **A C D E**
Conditions associated with abnormally wide fontanelles include rickets, hypothyroidism, cranio-synostosis and syndromes such as Smith-Lemli-Opitz, Zellweger's and Rubenstein-Tabyi.

17. **A B C D E**
Drugs such as alcohol and phenytoin cause ataxia in high levels.

Tumours such as cerebellar astrocytoma, pontine glioma and medulloblastoma can give rise to ataxia.

Neuroblastoma can give rise to dancing eye syndrome.

18. **A B**
Lennox-Gastaut syndrome consists of several different forms of epilepsy (atypical absences, axial tonic seizures and drop attacks), EEG changes of slow spike and wave when awake and 10 Hz bursts when asleep, and psychomotor retardation.

The condition often requires a combination of anticonvulsants to effect satisfactory treatment.

Only 4-6% of cases are self remitting, with poor prognostic factors including preceding developmental delay, neurological abnormality, or West's syndrome (infantile spasms). Early onset such as before 3 years of age, recurrent status epilepticus, poor fit control and slow background activity are also poor prognostic indicators.

19. **A B C D E**
Blindness in one eye may be due to retinal involvement as in a unilateral tumour, eg. due to an optic glioma. Atrophy may also give rise to unilateral blindness as in raised intracranial pressure.

Bitemporal hemianopia is characteristically seen in pituitary tumours with suprastellar involvement of the optic tracts or due to pressure effects on the optic chiasma.

Homonymous hemianopia may be due to a lesion involving the optic tract or the optic radiations from both eyes in the temporal and parietal pathways before reaching the appropiate occipital loci.

The optic pathways fan out, with lesions in the temporal aspects causing an homonymous superior field defect and lesions in the parietal tracts causing an inferior field defect.

The pupillary response is dependent on an intact C3 pathway with intact fibres running to the lateral geniculate body and on to the midbrain.

20. **A B C D E**
Refsum's disease is characterised by retinitis pigmentosa and peripheral neuropathy.

Riley-Day syndrome is associated with areflexia, absent tear formation, hypotonia, recurrent infections, increased sweating and a high pain threshold.

Hypothyroidism is associated with delayed reflexes, whereas in spinal muscular atrophy there is a congenital defect of the anterior horn cell hence the reflex arc is interrupted.

Guillain-Barré presents with a centripetal motor dysfunction which may be progressive to involve respiratory muscles, when assisted ventilation may be required. Autonomic nervous dysfunction may also occur with labile blood pressure and arrhthymias being seen.

21. **ALL FALSE**
The incidence of febrile convulsions in infancy is 5-7% with the majority occurring in the age group 9-24 months. A focus of infection *must always* be sought. The longer the convulsion the greater the risk of recurrence.

22. **B C E**

Macrocephaly	*Microcephaly*
achondroplasia	congenital infection eg rubella
Canavan's disease	fetal alcohol syndrome
Tay-Sach's syndrome	Angelman syndrome
Alexander's disease	Cornelia de Lange syndrome
neurofibromatosis	maternal phenylketonuria
Hunter's/Hurler's syndrome	Rubinstein-Tabyi syndrome
osteopetrosis	Edward/Patau syndrome
Soto's syndrome	Williams' syndrome

CHILDHOOD DEVELOPMENT

1. **At 6 months of age a child will**

   - [ ] A sit supported
   - [ ] B lie prone with arms extended
   - [ ] C cruise
   - [ ] D say 2–3 words
   - [ ] E use a spoon

2. **By 3 years of age, a child's gross motor function is sufficiently developed to allow him/her to**

   - [ ] A walk easily on a straight line drawn on the floor
   - [ ] B skip with alternating feet
   - [ ] C walk alone up stairs with alternating feet
   - [ ] D walk down stairs with alternating feet
   - [ ] E stand on one foot with arms folded

3. **Children should have their hearing tested**

   - [ ] A following recovery from bacterial meningitis
   - [ ] B if they are not using intelligible speech by 24 months
   - [ ] C if they are not using frequent repetitive babble by 10 months
   - [ ] D if they demonstrate articulation defects at 21 months
   - [ ] E if there is parental suspicion about the child having hearing difficulties

4. **By the age of 9 months a child's social development will allow him/her to**

   - [ ] A distinguish strangers from familiar people
   - [ ] B play peek-a-boo behind his/her hands
   - [ ] C verbalize the need to go to the toilet
   - [ ] D put on hat and shoes
   - [ ] E have tantrums in order to gain attention

5. A 12-month-old child will

- ☐ A build a tower of 3 bricks after being shown
- ☐ B refer to self by name
- ☐ C hold a pencil with preferred hand using 2 fingers and thumb
- ☐ D hold and drink from a cup held by an adult
- ☐ E crawl up stairs

6. The following should cause concern about the development of communication skills:

- ☐ A no single words by 13 months
- ☐ B repetitive babble not present by 10 months
- ☐ C parental worries about the child's hearing
- ☐ D the absence of grammatical structure by 5 years
- ☐ E echolalia by 2 years

ANSWERS AND TEACHING NOTES : CHILDHOOD DEVELOPMENT

1. **A B**

   Cruising takes place at about 10–12 months onwards; a child is able to say about 2–3 words from 15 months and can use a spoon after 18 months.

   At 6 months of age abilities are:

Gross motor skills	Supine raises head from pillow to gaze at feet
	Pulls to sit and stays sitting momentarily
	Rolls over front to back
	Prone lifts up head with shoulder girdle supported by extended arms
Vision and fine motor skills	Readily follows objects
	Uses palmar grasp and transfers
	Visual inattention if object rolls out of view
Hearing and speech	Recognises parental voice
	Babbles, laughs and gurgles with play
	Screams when annoyed
	Distraction testing for hearing normal
Social skills	Mouths and transfers objects
	Shakes rattle if offered
	Shy with strangers from 7 months

2. **C**

   Walking along a straight line with ease, standing on one leg with arms folded, skipping with alternating feet, hopping 2–3 yards forwards are all features of the 5-year-old child whereas at 3 years of age, he/she can walk up the stairs with alternating feet but comes down them two feet to a step. By 5 years of age the child should be able to walk forwards, backwards, sideways and has a good understanding of his/her own body space. The child should also be able to ride a tricycle by using the pedals and can direct it. She/he can stand and walk on tiptoe and will briefly stand on one foot when shown.

3. **A C E**

   Any children known to be at risk of deafness such as following bacterial meningitis or a strong family history must have their hearing checked. Any parental doubt must also lead to the hearing being tested.

   Other **indications for hearing investigation** include:
   - (i) failure to respond to surrounding noises or sounds by 6–8 weeks
   - (ii) absence of interest in people and toys by 3–4 months
   - (iii) absence of babble by 10 months
   - (iv) no single words by 21 months
   - (v) inability to put 2 or 3 words together by 2½ months
   - (vi) no intelligible speech by 4 years
   - (vii) absence of conventional grammatical language by 5 years
   - (viii) articulation defects at 6½ years.

Answers and Teaching Notes: Childhood Development

4. **A B**

   The last three answers fit with the social behaviour of a 2 year old. At this age, the child tends to be clingy to his parent, to throw tantrums in order to gain attention, to be possessive of toys and not to have yet learnt how to share toys.

   At 9 months the child can differentiate between strangers and those people known to him. He will try to grasp at the spoon when being fed and will use his hands to play games such as peek-a-boo and will clap his hands with vigour. Mouthing still occurs at this age.

5. **E**

   The ages appropriate for each question are:
   A at about 18 months
   B at about 2 years
   C at about 2 years
   D at about 15 months

   At 12 months of age, children are able to sit unsupported on the floor for an indefinite time, crawl on hands and knees, pull to stand and start to cruise. Some children can walk if held by the hand.

   The fine motor function at this time includes picking up 'hundreds and thousands', throwing toys and watching them fall and pointing to objects of interest. Hand preference may start at this time. Children will hold two bricks at the same time and bang them together. Hearing and speech development includes responding to name, babbling with vowels and consonants being used, and giving on request objects such as spoon, shoe etc.

   Distraction testing is limited as children tend to cotton on quite quickly!

   Social skills include holding a spoon but not being able to use it properly, putting objects in and out of boxes, giving toys on command to an adult. Children this age laugh and play with people well known to them.

6. **B C D**

   The failure of children to say single words at 21 months should raise concern. Echolalia may be normal at 2 years.

   The absence of grammatically correct sentences is a concern at 5 years and note of the domestic linguistic situation should be made.

   All children who are at risk of deafness or who have a strong family history of deafness should be screened at some point in childhood.

   Other worrying signs include:
   little or no response to surrounding sounds by 6–8 weeks
   an absence of interest in people and toys by 3–4 months
   failure of 2–3 word constructions by 27 months
   unintelligible speech by 4 years.

OPHTHALMOLOGY

1. **The following conditions may be complicated by congenital glaucoma:**

   - [ ] A Treacher-Collins syndrome
   - [ ] B neurofibromatosis I
   - [ ] C achondroplasia
   - [ ] D neurofibromatosis II
   - [ ] E Sturge-Weber syndrome

2. **Ophthalmia neonatorum**

   - [ ] A is most commonly caused by gonnorrhoea
   - [ ] B is a benign condition
   - [ ] C is a notifiable disease
   - [ ] D can be caused by chemical irritation
   - [ ] E if identified maternal high vaginal swabs must be taken

3. **The following conditions are associated with cataracts:**

   - [ ] A CHARGE syndrome
   - [ ] B Down's syndrome
   - [ ] C congenital rubella syndrome
   - [ ] D Zellweger syndrome
   - [ ] E phenylketonuria

4. **The following conditions are associated with colobomata of the iris:**

   - [ ] A VATER syndrome
   - [ ] B Turner's syndrome
   - [ ] C CHARGE syndrome
   - [ ] D septo-optic dysplasia
   - [ ] E Cruzon syndrome

5. Squints

- [ ] A are easily correctable
- [ ] B may be corrected by patching
- [ ] C can lead to amblyopia
- [ ] D can be associated with an underlying lesion
- [ ] E may be misdiagnosed in the presence of epicanthic folds

ANSWERS AND TEACHING NOTES : OPHTHALMOLOGY

1. **A B D E**
   Both types of neurofibromatosis, Treacher-Collins syndrome and Sturge-Weber syndrome can lead to congenital glaucoma or busophthalmos and blindness if not treated appropriately. Other causative conditions are retinoblastoma, Zellweger syndrome, Marfan syndrome, homocystinuria, fetal rubella effects and in the aniridia-Wilms' tumour association.

2. **C D E**
   Ophthalmia neonatorum refers to any chronic discharge from a baby's eyes in the first month of life. It is a notifiable condition and is definitely not benign. Gonorrhoea is no longer the commonest cause of ophthalmia neonatorum in developed countries. Chlamydia is probably the commonest infective cause with onset between 4–14 days of life. Overall chemical irritation in the developed world is the highest offender, examples are use of silver nitrates. The condition must be appropriately treated to avoid irreversible damage and the possible maternal source investigated and treated.

3. **B C D**
   The following conditions are associated with cataracts:
   Down's syndrome
   congenital rubella syndrome
   Zellweger syndrome
   Cockayne syndrome
   aniridia-Wilms' tumour association
   Incontinentia Pigmenti
   Rubinstein-Taybi syndrome
   Turner's syndrome
   nail-patella syndrome

4. **C D E**
   The following conditions are associated with colobomata of the iris:
   CHARGE syndrome
   septo-optic dysplasia
   Cruzon syndrome
   aniridia-Wilms' tumour association
   Marfan syndrome
   linear sebaceous neavus sequence
   Rubinstein-Taybi syndrome
   Sturge-Weber syndrome.

5. **C D E**
   Squints are extremely common and vary markedly in their severity and correction with surgery. Patching is carried out if concerns about a 'lazy eye' develop and there is risk of amblyopia. Squints may

occasionally be misdiagnosed in the presence of epicanthic folds such as occur in Down's syndrome. Great care should always be taken to ensure that there is not an underlying lesion interfering with eye movement.

RHEUMATOLOGY/ORTHOPAEDICS

1. **Systemic rheumatoid arthritis**

   ☐ A invariably demonstrates a low ESR
   ☐ B occurs mainly in boys above 5 years
   ☐ C rarely occurs before 5 years
   ☐ D is associated with neutropenia
   ☐ E is associated with antinuclear antibodies

2. **Polyarthritic IgM rheumatoid factor positive arthritis**

   ☐ A has a male preponderance
   ☐ B usually occurs after 8 years of age
   ☐ C is associated with formation of rheumatoid nodules on pressure points
   ☐ D is not associated with vasculitis
   ☐ E is associated with HLA DR4

3. **Pauciarticular rheumatoid arthritis of younger onset**

   ☐ A requires onset below 6 years to fit this classification
   ☐ B is more common in boys
   ☐ C carries a high risk of chronic iridocyclitis
   ☐ D is frequently associated with HLA B27
   ☐ E is associated with antinuclear antibodies

4. **Juvenile psoriatic arthritis is associated with**

   ☐ A a preponderance of affected females
   ☐ B symmetrical arthritis
   ☐ C presence of IgM rheumatoid factor
   ☐ D the occasional presence of antinuclear antibodies
   ☐ E iridocyclitis

5. Reactive arthritis in children

- A includes Reiter's syndrome
- B does not occur before puberty
- C is most common in males
- D is associated with a high ESR
- E is often associated with HLA B27

6. Perthes' disease

- A usually occurs over 10 years of age
- B is more common in girls
- C is more common in obese children
- D requires internal fixation of the hip
- E can be bilateral

7. Osteogenesis imperfecta type I

- A is inherited in an autosomal recessive manner
- B is associated with childhood kyphoscoliosis
- C leads to an increased fracture rate in adolescence
- D is associated with hearing defects after ten years of age in most cases
- E is not associated with blue sclera

8. Osteogenesis imperfecta type III

- A results in stillbirth in 50% of cases
- B is of X-linked recessive inheritance
- C classically is associated with intrauterine growth retardation
- D cases often have wormian bones on skull X-ray
- E is associated with blue sclera at birth which gradually becomes less marked

9. Congenital talipes equinovarus

- [ ] A occurs in about 1 in 100 live births
- [ ] B has a sex ratio of 1 male to 2 females
- [ ] C results in the foot being inverted and supinated with the forefoot adducted
- [ ] D does not respond to manipulation
- [ ] E may have oligohydramnios as a factor

10. Hemihypertrophy may be associated with

- [ ] A Wilms' tumour
- [ ] B neurofibromata
- [ ] C haemangioma
- [ ] D lymphangioma
- [ ] E otitis externa

11. Congenital dislocation of the hip

- [ ] A affects more boys than girls
- [ ] B has a lower incidence in children born by caesarian section
- [ ] C has a higher incidence in premature babies
- [ ] D has a risk of 1 in 15 for first degree female relatives
- [ ] E if present can always be picked up by examination

12. These conditions are lethal forms of dysplasia:

- [ ] A Ellis-van Creveld syndrome
- [ ] B thanatophoric dwarfism
- [ ] C asphyxiating thoracic dystrophy
- [ ] D homozygous achondroplasia
- [ ] E osteogenesis imperfecta type II

13. Causes of torticollis include

- [ ] A cervical adenitis
- [ ] B posterior fossa tumour
- [ ] C Poland's anomaly
- [ ] D Klippel-Feil syndrome
- [ ] E IV nerve palsy

ANSWERS AND TEACHING NOTES : RHEUMATOLOGY/ORTHOPAEDICS

1. **ALL FALSE**

   Systemic rheumatoid arthritis usually occurs before 5 years of age, being of equal incidence during this period. Onset after 5 years is commoner in girls.

   Clinical features include high remittent fever, myalgia, malaise, salmon pink/red maculopapular rash, lymphadenopathy, hepatosplenomegaly, serositis (especially pericarditis), hepatitis, progressive anaemia and arthritis (knees, wrists and carpi, ankles and tarsi, neck, followed by other joints).

   Investigations reveal high ESR, low Hb, neutrophil leucocytosis, thrombocythaemia, IgM -ve and antinuclear antibodies -ve.

2. **B C E**
   Polyarthritic rheumatoid arthritis

	IgM RhF -ve	*IgM RhF +ve*
Age of onset	Any age	Over 8 years
Sex preponderance	Female	Female
Joints affected	Any joint	Any joint
	Especially knees, wrists, ankles and P/DIP joints of hands. MCP often spared.	Small joints of the wrist, hands, ankles and feet. Knees and hips early involvement, with elbows later.
Other specific features	Limitation of neck and temporomandibular movement. Flexor tenosynovitis, low-grade fever, occasional mild lymphadenopathy and hepatosplenomegaly.	Rheumatoid nodules on pressure points, especially elbows. Vasculitis (uncommon and often late), nail fold lesion and ulceration.
ESR	Raised	Usually raised
Hb	Occasionally down	Moderate anaemia
WBC	Mild neutrophil leucocytosis	–
Platelets	Moderate thrombocytosis	–
ANA	Occasionally +ve	Occasionally +ve
HLA association	–	DR4

Answers and Teaching Notes: Rheumatology/Orthopaedics

3. **A C E**
   Pauciarticular rheumatoid arthritis refers to a condition with involvement of four joints or less.

Type	Younger	Older
Age	< 6 years	> 6 years
Sex	More common in females	More common in males
Clinical features	Commonly knee, ankle, elbow or a single finger joint. Poor growth. 1 in 3 risk of chronic iridocyclitis in first 5 years of the disease.	Peripheral arthritis, predominantly lower limb joints. Enthesiophathies, plantar fascia, Achilles tendon. Occasional sacroiliac pain and axial disease.
ESR	N/raised	N/raised
Fbc	N	N
IgM RhF	–ve	–ve
ANA	Frequently +ve	–ve
HLA status	A2, DR5, DRw6 and DRw8	B27

4. **A D E**
   Juvenile psoriatic arthritis is associated with a typical psoriatic rash and an arthritis occurring at the same time or separately. Further there is dactylitis, nail pitting and often a family history of psoriasis. The condition is more common in females. Clinically the arthritis is classically asymmetrical, flexor tenosynovitis occurs and occasionally the condition may lead to severe destructive disease.

   ESR varies with the number of joints affected and accordingly may be very high, Hb is occasionally low, WBC can rise, IgM RhF is –ve and antinuclear antibodies are occasionally present.

   Onset in younger children may be complicated by development of iridocyclitis.

5. **A C D E**
   Reactive arthritis tends to occur after an intercurrent infection without evidence of the causative organism in the joint. It is found at any age, but particularly after puberty. There is a male preponderance. Clinical features include arthritis, urethritis, balanitis, cystitis, conjunctivitis (all associated with Reiter's syndrome), mouth ulcers, fever and rashes (including keratoderma blennorrhagia). ESR is usually high, WBC shows mild polymorph leucocytosis, Hb is normal, IgM RhF is –ve, there are no antinuclear antibodies. Occasionally there are positive stool or urethral cultures (*Shigella, Salmonella, Yersinia, Campylobacter, Chlamydia*). There is a high incidence of HLA B27.

Answers and Teaching Notes: Rheumatology/Orthopaedics

6. **C E**
Perthes' disease is an inflammatory disorder of the hips, being either unilateral or bilateral, occurring most often in obese boys between 5–10 years of age. The cause is unknown. The condition usually settles with bed rest, limited physiotherapy, simple analgesics and occasionally traction. It is unusual for more aggressive therapy to be necessary.

7. **D**
Osteogenesis imperfecta type I is the most common form, being of autosomal dominant inheritance and consisting of osteoporosis, excessive bone fragility, distinct blue sclera and presenile conductive hearing loss in adolescents and adults. Clinically there is bowing of the lower limbs and 20% of adults are found to have a progressive kyphoscoliosis. This a rare finding in childhood. There is excessive laxity of ligaments, especially small joints, which becomes less marked with age. The frequency of spontaneous fractures decreases from adolescence onwards.

8. **D E**
Osteogenesis imperfecta type III is a severe condition resulting in bone fragility and multiple fracture. However stillbirth and intrauterine growth retardation are features of the even more severe type II form. The sclera are blue at birth but become less so with age. Inheritance is autosomal recessive. Children develop kyphoscoliosis and final stature is short. Hearing impairment is not a problem. Skull X-rays may demonstrate the classical wormian bone appearance. Death tends to be in infancy or early childhood from cardiorespiratory complications.

9. **C E**
This condition occurs about 1 in 1000 births with a sex ratio of two males to every female. Manipulation should be used as early as possible and severe cases should be referred to an orthopaedic surgeon.

Implicated factors in the development of this condition include oligohydramnios and abnormal intrauterine positioning.

10. **A B C D**
This condition may be very subtle with the only findings being that the limbs are slightly thicker unilaterally, there are differing amounts of hair on opposite parts of the body or there is a variation in eruption and size of teeth.

The relative difference is maintained with the proportions growing at uniform rates throughout physical growth.

11. **D**
The overall incidence of congenital dislocation of the hip is 1.25 per 1000 live births. The incidence is six times higher in girls than in

Answers and Teaching Notes: Rheumatology/Orthopaedics

boys and the left hip is more often involved than the right. The risk to first degree males is 1 in 100, with an increased frequency of occurence in babies born by breech extraction. The incidence is not altered in babies born by Caesarian section. Premature babies have a lower incidence possibly due to the absence of joint-relaxing maternal hormones.

12. B C D E

Ellis-van Creveld syndrome is characterised by skeletal defects, in particular shortening of the long bones distal to the elbow and the knees, with the thorax being narrow and short. The face and head, bones of the vertebrae and pelvis are normal. There are commonly ectodermal anomalies of teeth, nails and hair. The teeth tend to be small and peg like. The nails may be hypoplastic or absent. There is fine sparse hair. 50% of cases have congenital heart disease, the majority of these being an atrial septal defect. IQ is unimpaired.

Thanatophoric dwarfism is a lethal condition with shortened limbs and thorax. The head appears large in relation to the body and often shows a prominent forehead. The cause of death is usually marked respiratory distress within the neonatal period.

Asphyxiating thoracic dystrophy of jeune is a lethal abnormality owing to a failure of ossification of costochondral cartilage. This leads to a narrow bell-shaped chest which fails to develop with the child's growth. Hence, death arises due to respiratory insufficiency. In association there may be pulmonary hypoplasia.

Homozygous achondroplasia is a lethal condition arising from the conjunction of two parents with achondroplasia. Again death tends to occur within the neonatal period. The child has a characteristic large cranium, small chest and short limbs.

Osteogenesis imperfecta encompasses a number of types of 'fragile' bone disorders with varying modes of inheritance. The most lethal form is osteogenesis lethalis or type II when the baby is stillborn or dies within the neonatal period. Type I is the commonest form associated with blue sclera and fractures generally occurring when the child is a toddler. Deafness caused by otosclerosis is commonly seen. In type III, which is an autosomal recessive condition, fractures appear from the neonatal period onwards. This disorder is associated with limb deformity and shortening. Deafness is unusual in this condition. Type IV is inherited in a dominant fashion but the sclera are generally of normal colour. Fractures again occur from birth; however, this condition does not produce as marked limb shortening as type III.

13. A B D E

Muscular causes include congenital sternoclediomastoid tumour, trauma and local inflammation as in cervical lymphadenopathy.

Ocular causes such as IVth nerve palsy, brain stem tumours or posterior fossa tumours with a VIth lesion with the torticollis being performed so as to overcome the visual effect of the concomitant squint.

Vertebral anomalies such as fusion of vertebrae as in Klippel-Feil anomaly of the upper cervical vertebrae, hemi vertebrae or Sprengel's shoulder may be associated with torticollis.

INFECTIOUS DISEASES

1. **The incubation times for the following diseases are true:**

   - [ ] A chickenpox has a minimum incubation time of 5 weeks
   - [ ] B mumps has an incubation period of 1 week
   - [ ] C rubella can present by 2 weeks
   - [ ] D measles has an incubation time of up to 2 weeks
   - [ ] E hepatitis A can take 5 weeks to present

2. **These conditions are notifiable in England and Wales:**

   - [ ] A hepatitis B
   - [ ] B influenza
   - [ ] C mumps
   - [ ] D rubella
   - [ ] E meningococcaemia

3. *Listeria monocytogenes*

   - [ ] A is a Gram-negative rod
   - [ ] B is found intracellularly
   - [ ] C is capable of surviving 'cook–chill' techniques for food preparation
   - [ ] D can give rise to hepatosplenomegaly in neonates
   - [ ] E may present at 1–4 weeks after delivery with meningitis

4. **Anthrax**

   - [ ] A is a Gram-negative encapsulated spore-forming nonmotile rod
   - [ ] B is transmissable by contact with infected hides
   - [ ] C gives rise to Eschar(s) in the cutaneous form
   - [ ] D has an incubation period of 3 months
   - [ ] E can be diagnosed by fluorescent antibody testing of the organism from vesicular fluid

Infectious Diseases

5. **Rubella**

   ☐ A can cause congenital rubella syndrome if primary maternal infection occurs at 18 weeks' gestation
   ☐ B prodromal period is about 14–21 days
   ☐ C rash may be confused with parvovirus rash
   ☐ D in the congenital form, may present with an interstitial pneumonitis
   ☐ E in congenital syndrome most often causes ventricular defects

6. **Toxoplasmosis occurring in pregnancy may cause the following in the neonate:**

   ☐ A hydrops fetalis
   ☐ B pneumonitis
   ☐ C microphthalmia
   ☐ D ocular lesions which may be delayed in onset as late as school age or older
   ☐ E congenital adrenal hypoplasia

7. *Bacillus cereus*

   ☐ A has an incubation period of 3 days
   ☐ B is transmitted by direct contact from person to person
   ☐ C is a Gram-positive spore-forming organism
   ☐ D produces an exotoxin
   ☐ E always requires systemic antibiotics

8. *Mycoplasma pneumoniae*

   ☐ A can give rise to an aseptic meningitis
   ☐ B causes a haemolytic anaemia
   ☐ C can be transmitted from infected birds
   ☐ D has an incubation period of 2 weeks
   ☐ E is a Gram-positive organism with a double cell wall

9. **The following are RNA viruses or are caused by RNA viruses:**

   ☐ A molluscum contagiosum
   ☐ B parvovirus
   ☐ C Epstein-Barr
   ☐ D adenovirus
   ☐ E measles

10. **Diagnostic criteria for Kawasaki disease include**

    ☐ A a 2-day history of pyrexia
    ☐ B an acute arthritis
    ☐ C inguinal lymphadenopathy alone
    ☐ D hepatosplenomegaly
    ☐ E a polymorphous rash

11. **Poor prognostic indicators for meningococcaemia at presentation include**

    ☐ A meningism
    ☐ B low white cell count
    ☐ C normal clotting indices
    ☐ D petechiae present for more than 12 hours
    ☐ E normal ESR

12. **Adenovirus**

    ☐ A causes a tonsillitis
    ☐ B causes acute otitis media
    ☐ C is the commonest single aetiological agent for febrile convulsions
    ☐ D causes keratitis
    ☐ E causes 10–20% of pneumonia seen in childhood

13. Common causative organisms for septic arthritis in the UK include

- [ ] A *Pseudomonas*
- [ ] B *Klebsiella*
- [ ] C *Actinomyces*
- [ ] D *Candida*
- [ ] E *Cryptococcus*

14. The following are indicative of paediatric AIDS:

- [ ] A oral candidiasis
- [ ] B generalized dermatitis
- [ ] C disseminated *Mycobacterium kansasii*
- [ ] D cytomegalovirus retinitis
- [ ] E chronic intestinal cryptosporosis

15. *Borrelia burgdorferi*

- [ ] A is a Gram-positive diplococcus
- [ ] B causes an aseptic meningitis
- [ ] C gives a positive VDRL result
- [ ] D can be treated with penicillin
- [ ] E requires the eradication of fresh water snails to prevent its spread

ANSWERS AND TEACHING NOTES : INFECTIOUS DISEASES

1. **C D E**

	Incubation times in days	
	Average	Ranges
Chickenpox	14	7–14
Measles	10	7–14
Mumps	17	14–21
Rubella	17	14–21
Hepatitis A	28	14–70
Hepatitis B	60	40–160
Fifth's disease	7	3–14
Diphtheria	21	14–21
Infectious mononucleosis	28	14–56
Whooping cough	10	7–14

2. **A C D E**
   The current **list of notifiable diseases** comprises:

Acute encephalitis	Meningococcaemia	Viral haemorrhage
Acute polio	Mumps	Viral hepatitis
Anthrax	Neonatal ophthalmia	Whooping cough
Cholera	Paratyphoid	Yellow fever
Diphtheria	Plague	
Dysentery	Rabies	
Food poisoning	Rubella	
Leprosy	Scarlet fever	
Leptospirosis	Smallpox	
Malaria	Tetanus	
Measles	Tuberculosis	
Meningitis	Typhoid fever	

3. **A B C D E**

   Listeria monocytogenes is a Gram-positive rod, which can cause disease in the elderly, immunosuppressed and pregnant women. It grows intracellularly and can survive the 'cook–chill' methods of food preparation. It has also been grown from soft cheeses, particularly in endemic areas of France and Switzerland, from paté and from poorly cooked meats.

   In the pregnant woman it may cause a febrile illness, with a sore throat and headache, and transplacental passage infection of the neonate may occur.

   After delivery the baby may develop respiratory distress syndrome, apnoea, convulsions and have hepatosplenomegaly. There are characteristic pin-point granulomata, particularly seen on the face. About a third of these neonates also have meningitis due to the organism.

   A later onset of infection by *Listeria* is also seen. This occurs from 1 week of life onwards up to 4 weeks of age with the majority of these cases presenting with meningitis.

Answers and Teaching Notes : Infectious Diseases

4. **B C E**
Anthrax is caused by *Bacillus anthracis*, a Gram-positive encapsulated spore forming organism which is nonmotile. Spores can lie dormant in soil or in infected tissues such as hides for several years. The commonest manifestation is the cutaneous form which is associated with Eschar formation. Pulmonary and gastro-intestinal infection also occur and may have a fatal course by way of septicaemia and/or meningitis.

The incubation period is 1–7 days with most cases occurring within 2–5 days of exposure.

Diagnostic tests include microscope identification on Gram staining, fluorescent antibody directed against the organism in infected tissue, antibody elevation to *Bacillus anthracis* toxin by immunoblot or rise in serum antibody by ELISA test in acute and convalescent samples.

5. **C D**
The risk of congenital rubella syndrome before 11 weeks' gestation is about 90% whereas sensorineural deafness tends to occur if the fetus is affected between 11–16 weeks. After this time the risk to the fetus is very low.

5–20 % of women of child-bearing age are non-immune, with transplacental primary infection and to a much smaller extent reinfection being the causes of congenital rubella syndrome.

Reinfections with rubella can occur in pregnancy and are often subclinical with a rise in IgG titres. Replication of rubella can take place and transplacental infection may arise.

Rubelliform rashes may be seen with parvovirus, particularly with B19 infection and are also noted in enterovirus infection.

Features of congenital rubella syndrome:

Ophthalmic	congenital cataracts
	choroidoretinitis
	microphthalmia
CNS	microcephaly
	panencephalitis
	sensorineural deafness
Respiratory	interstitial pneumonitis
Reticular endothelial	splenomegaly
	hepatomegaly
	thrombocytopenia
CVS	pulmonary stenosis
	patent ductus arteriosus
	coarctation of the aorta
Renal	polycystic kidneys
	renal artery stenosis

Endocrine	diabetes mellitus
thyroid disease
growth hormone deficiency
precocious puberty

The diagnosis may be made on raised specific IgM titres from the cord or neonatal blood or by direct culture of virus from nasopharyngeal secretions, from eye swabs, urine or stool.

6. **A B C D**
   Congenital toxoplasmosis, caused by the protozoan *T. gondii* affects 1–7 per 1000 live births.

   There may be systemic involvement such as:
   hydrops fetalis
   thrombocytopenia
   dermal erythropoiesis
   hepatosplenomegaly
   lymphadenopathy
   pneumonitis

   CNS involvement:
   fits
   nystagmus
   choroidoretinitis
   cataracts
   microcephaly
   hydrocephaly

   The diagnosis is made by finding raised specific IgM in cord or neonatal blood.

7. **C D**
   Bacillus cereus is a Gram-positive spore forming organism (but can live as a facultative anaerobe) and may produce two clinical types of food poisoning.

   One form has a short incubation period of 1–6 hours with vomiting, nausea and diarrhoea being the key features of an exotoxin which is liberated.

   The second form has a longer incubation period of up to 16 hours. The clinical manifestations of this condition include abdominal cramps and diarrhoea. This is thought to be due to an enterotoxin being released from the cell wall.

   Supportive treatment is usually all that is required in food posioning due to *Bacillus cereus*.

Answers and Teaching Notes : Infectious Diseases

8. **A B D**
    This is an organism without a cell wall with man as the only source of infection. The incubation period is 2–3 weeks and infection may manifest as an upper respiratory tract infection, otitis media, aseptic meningitis, encephalitis, peripheral neuropathy, myocarditis, Stevens-Johnson syndrome and a haemolytic anaemia due to cold agglutination disease.

9. **E**
    The following are **DNA containing viruses**:
Poxvirus	(eg. variola, vaccinia, molluscum contagiosum)
Herpesvirus	(eg. Herpes simplex, varicella, Epstein-Barr and cytomegalovirus)
Adenovirus	Many serotypes
Parvovirus	Fifth disease

    The following are RNA viruses:
Orthomyxovirus	Influenza A, B and C
Paramyxovirus	Parainfluenza, measles
Togavirus	Yellow fever, dengue
Picornavirus	Enterovirus which includes polio, echo, rotavirus
Retrovirus	HTLV-I,II
	HIV-I,II

10. **E**
    Diagnostic criteria for Kawasaki:
    1. Pyrexia of unknown origin for at least 5 days
    2. The presence of 4 out of these 5 conditions:
        (i) cervical lymphadenopathy
        (ii) polymorphous rash
        (iii) bilateral injection of conjunctiva
        (iv) changes in mucous membranes: reddened pharynx, swollen lips, strawberry tongue
        (v) changes in palms/soles: oedema, erythema or later desquamation
    3. Exclusion of other illnesses such as staphylococcal, streptococcal infection, Stevens-Johnson syndrome, measles, leptospirosis and ricketsial infections. Collagen disorders such as juvenile rheumatoid arthritis must also be excluded.

    In the presence of coronary aneurysms, only (i) and (iii) out of the conditions in section 2 are required to make a diagnosis.

11. **B E**
    Mortality rates are greater than 90% in patients with three or more of the following:
    – petechial rash of less than 12 hours

- shock
- peripheral white cell count of less than $10 \times 10^9/1$
- low or normal ESR.

12. A B C D E
Adenovirus accounts for 5–8% of respiratory infections in childhood and can cause aseptic meningitis, encephalitis, diarrhoea and hepatitis. These are non-enveloped DNA viruses, grouped into six subsera A–F by serology and DNA typing.

Most commonly they cause infection between the age of 6 months and 5 years, by direct contact, by aerosol or by the faecal-oral route. Outbreaks occur in close knit communities. The diagnosis can be confirmed by viral culture, antigen detection or by serology.

13. ALL FALSE
Common organisms causing septic arthritis are:
- *Staphylococcus aureus*
- Gram-negative enteric bacteria
- *Haemophilius influenzae*
- *Streptococcus*
- *Pneumococcus*
- gonococci
- meningococci
- *Salmonella*.

14. C D E
Diagnoses which are indicative of AIDS include:
Candidasis of the oesophagus, trachea, bronchi or lungs
Coccidiomycosis, disseminated
Cryptococcosis, extrapulmonary
Cryptosporosis, chronic intestinal
Cytomegalovirus disease onset at age 1 month or retinitis (excluding liver, spleen or lymph nodes)
Herpes simplex, chronic ulcer, pneumonitis, oesophagitis
Histoplasmosis, extrapulmonary or disseminated
Kaposi's sarcoma
Lymphoid interstitial pneumonitis
Lymphoma, primary brain
Mycobacterium avium/kansasii disseminated or extrapulmonary
Pneumocystis carinii pneumonia
Toxoplasmosis, cerebral onset after 1 month of age.

15. B D

Borrelia burgdorferi is a spirochaete transmitted by ticks of the genus Ioxodes (this genus includes the deer tick, the commonest vector for Lyme disease transmission) and causes Lyme disease. The early manifestations are a red macular-papular rash which expands whilst retaining a central paler zone close to the site of the tick bite. This may extend, becoming known as erythema chronicum migrans.

Fever, malaise and arthralgia may occur intermittently over a few weeks.

Secondary manifestations may be seen after a few months such as joint involvement, ocular disorders, CNS and cardiac involvement including carditis, cranial nerve palsies and aseptic meningitis.

The incubation period is 3 to 35 days.

Serological testing is most commonly used to confirm the diagnosis as the spirochaetes are not often cultured.

ELISA testing and an indirect fluorescent antibody test are available. Western blotting has also been developed.

IgM titres rise between 3–6 weeks after infection whilst IgG titres rise more slowly taking months to become elevated. Antibodies to *Borrelia burgdorferi* may cross react with other spirochaetes such as *Treponema pallidum* but patients affected with Lyme disease do not produce positive VDRL results.

Treatment in childhood in the early stages of the disease includes penicillin, amoxycillin or erythromycin. In adults, tetracycline may be used.

DERMATOLOGY

1. These lesions are seen in tuberous sclerosis:

   ☐ A pyoderma gangrenosum
   ☐ B molluscum contagiosum
   ☐ C indurated areas of skin, particularly on the back
   ☐ D erythema nodosum
   ☐ E hypopigmented patches

2. The following lesions may become malignant conditions:

   ☐ A milia
   ☐ B neuroma
   ☐ C spider naevi
   ☐ D hyperkeratosis
   ☐ E alopecia areata

3. Patients with diabetes mellitus may demonstrate:

   ☐ A cutaneous candidiasis
   ☐ B necrobiosis lipoidica
   ☐ C granuloma annulare
   ☐ D lipoatrophy
   ☐ E eruptive xanthoma

4. Psoriasis

   ☐ A commonly presents in guttate form in childhood
   ☐ B may present solely with onycholysis
   ☐ C is associated with peripheral arthropathy in over 80% of cases in childhood
   ☐ D in the pustular presentation affecting the palms and soles is seen in 40% of cases
   ☐ E affecting the scalp can resemble seborrhoea

Dermatology

5. Photosensitivity is seen in

- [ ] A xeroderma pigmentosum
- [ ] B Bloom's syndrome
- [ ] C Cockayne's syndrome
- [ ] D Hartnup's disease
- [ ] E papular acrodermatitis

6. Atopic eczema

- [ ] A is seen in the majority of affected patients by 6 months of age
- [ ] B is exacerbated by superadded infection with herpes simplex
- [ ] C has an increased tendency to form IgE antibody to inhalants and foods
- [ ] D is poorly correlated to the development of allergic rhinitis
- [ ] E can become lichenified

7. Hypopigmentation is seen with

- [ ] A Waardenburg's syndrome
- [ ] B hypomelanosis of Ito
- [ ] C *Candida albicans*
- [ ] D tinea versicolor
- [ ] E scarlet fever

8. The following are true:

- [ ] A alopecia areata is due to *Trichophyton* infection
- [ ] B trichillomania gives rise to repeated areas of scarring
- [ ] C exclamation hairs are seen with scalp involvement of SLE
- [ ] D invariably hair loss from mechanical traction at assisted deliveries is permanent
- [ ] E traction alopecia may be associated with follicular pustules

Dermatology

9. The following are causes of erythema nodosum:

- ☐ A *Mycobacterium leprosum*
- ☐ B streptococcal infection
- ☐ C tuberculosis
- ☐ D *Mycoplasma pneumoniae*
- ☐ E histoplasmosis

10. Erythema toxicum

- ☐ A has a mortality of 50%
- ☐ B occurs most commonly in the first 24–48 hours of life
- ☐ C may herald a widespread vasculitis
- ☐ D will demonstrate eosinophils from pustules under microscopy
- ☐ E most commonly resolves after infancy

ANSWERS AND TEACHING NOTES : DERMATOLOGY

1. **C E**
   Cutaneous manifestations of tuberous sclerosis include shagreen patches which are indurated areas of skin often on the back in the lower lumbar or sacral region. Ashleaf patches are areas of hypopigmentation and subungal fibromata. Angiofibromas appear as 2–4mm bright erythematous papules. These were formerly known as adenoma subaceum and are a distinctive feature.

2. **B**
   Neuroma associated with neurofibromatosis may undergo malignant change. The other conditions do not undergo malignant change.

3. **A B C D E**
   There is an increased susceptibility for cutaneous candidiasis to arise in diabetes mellitus.
   Necrobiosis lipoidica appears as a sharply marginated yellow or brownish-yellow area of shiny atrophic skin.
   Granuloma annulare has the appearance of a serpingous elevated lesion with a clearly demarcated edge. Some cases have been seen after exposure to sun.
   Eruptive xanthoma may also occur in liver disease, myxoedema and chronic pancreatitis.
   Carotenaemia is also seen in diabetes, being a yellowish pigmentation of the palms of the hands and soles of the feet. Mild carotenaemia is also reported in hypothyroidism and some forms of hyperlipidaemia.

4. **A B**
   Arthropathy is uncommon in childhood as is involvement of the palms and soles.
   Guttate psoriasis is a common presentation, with the eruptions often preceded by an upper respiratory tract infection.
   Nail involvement may be the only manifestation with onycholysis and salmon patches being seen.

5. **A B C D**
   Xeroderma pigmentosum is due to a genetic defect in repairing DNA damaged by ultra-violet radiation hence blistering and cutaneous ulcers are seen. The incidence of cutaneous malignancies is increased in particular for basal cell and squamous cell carcinomas and malignant melanomas.
   Bloom's syndrome is an autosomal recessive disorder with a photosensitive rash, short stature and increased incidence of leukaemia, lymphoma and nephroblastoma. Immunoglobulin deficiencies are also seen giving rise to an increased incidence of respiratory or gastrointestinal infections.

Answers and Teaching Notes: Dermatology

Cockayne's syndrome is associated with short trunk and long limbs, along with mental delay, optic atrophy and cerebellar dysfunction.

Hartnup's disease is due to a defect in transport across the small bowel and the proximal renal tubules of the neutral amino acids. A pellagra-like rash occurs with exposure to the sun.

Papular acrodermatitis known as Gianotti Crosti syndrome is seen in pre-school children with discrete red papules in large quantities on the limbs. The rash resolves after 1 month.

Viruses which have been implicated in this syndrome include hepatitis B, hepatitis A, adenovirus, cytomegalovirus and rotavirus.

6. **A B C E**

Atopic eczema is a genetically predisposed condition typified by an increased tendency to form antibodies (particularly IgE) to foods and inhaled substances. About 75% of patients will have shown signs of eczema by 6 months of age and have an increased incidence of allergic conditions such as allergic rhinitis and asthma. The child presents with pruritus and dryness of the skin. With repeated scratching lichenification is seen.

The extent of involvement may be limited or may be generalised. The face and extensor surfaces are most commonly involved.

7. **A B D**

Waardenburg's syndrome is an autosomal dominantly inherited condition associated with a white forelock, sensorineural deafness and heterochromic irises. There may also be patches of hypopigmented macules and papules.

Hypomelanosis of Ito (also known as incontinentia pigmenti) may present with a marble like lesion running in linear streaks. These may appear blistered with a normal or decreased number of melanocytes. In contrast there are no inflammatory cells in the dermis. Associated with this disorder are musculoskeletal abnormalities, CNS abnormalities with fits, developmental delay and motor defects.

Tinea versicolor may vary in colour from dark brown to hypopigmented patches.

Common disorders of pigmentation include: pityriasis alba, vilitigo, tinea versicolor. Tuberous sclerosis may also have hypopigmentated patches and Ashleaf patches.

8. **E**

Trichophyton is the commonest fungal genus associated with tinea capitis. Trichillomania is associated with a patchy diffuse pattern of hair loss without the presence of scars and nail biting. There may be other evidence of dermatitis artifacta.

Exclamation hairs are characteristic of alopecia areata with tapered shafts of hair.

Any hair lost at delivery rapidly regrows, sadly fading in middle age!

Answers and Teaching Notes: Dermatology

Hair loss can also be seen following treatment with drugs such cytotoxic agents and with valproate.

Iron deficiency and hypothyoidism may also be associated with shedding of hair.

9. **A B C D E**
   Infective causes of erythema nodosum include:
   - Bacterial organisms such as streptococcal disease, meningococcal infection, tuberculosis, leprosy, psittacosis, and *Yersinia*
   - Fungal infections such as histoplasmosis, coccidiomycosis
   - Other organisms such as cat-scratch-fever, *Chlamydia*

   Note that systemic disorders such as sarcoidosis, ulcerative colitis and Crohn's disease may also cause erythema nodosum.

   Other agents such as drugs eg. sulphonamides and the combined oral contraceptive pill may cause erythema nodosum.

   Strictly speaking leprosy causes erythema nodosum leprosum which differs as it lasts a few days before complete resolution occurs.

10. **B D**
    Erythema toxicum (also known as urticaria neonatorum) is a benign self-limiting condition, appearing in the first few days of life and resolving in the majority of cases in the first 2 weeks of life. There is an associated peripheral eosinophilia and eosinophils if the fluid from the pustules is examined microscopically. Most commonly the lesions affect the face and trunk, less commonly affecting the palms or soles, with an appearance of a nettle rash.

GENETICS AND SYNDROMES

1. When considering the following family tree:

    Generation:

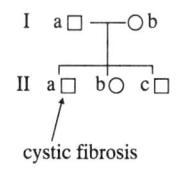

    I   a☐ ──── ○ b

    II a☐ b○ c☐
        ↑
    cystic fibrosis

    Carrier rate for cystic fibrosis is 1 in 25.

    ☐ A IIa should have genetic counselling as to the risk of his progeny having cystic fibrosis
    ☐ B IIb may be offered prenatal and antenatal testing for cystic fibrosis
    ☐ C IIb has a 1 in 2 chance of being affected
    ☐ D IIc has a 1 in 2 chance of being affected
    ☐ E children of IIc have a 1 in 150 chance of being affected

2. Genetic causes of blindness include

    ☐ A retrolental fibroplasia
    ☐ B birth asphyxia
    ☐ C cortical blindness
    ☐ D Leber's amaurosis
    ☐ E Lawrence-Moon-Biedl syndrome

3. The following are X-linked recessive disorders:

    ☐ A nephrogenic diabetes insipidus
    ☐ B vitamin D resistant rickets
    ☐ C ataxic telangiectasia
    ☐ D myotonia dystrophia
    ☐ E chronic granulomatous disease

4. The following are true for single-gene disorders:

    ☐ A in autosomal recessive conditions the risk to male offspring of female carriers is 1 in 2
    ☐ B in autosomal dominant conditions with full penetrance the risk to an affected individual that he/she might transmit the disorder to subsequent children is 1 in 4
    ☐ C in X-linked recessive disorders the parents are normal but the risk to daughters of carrier females being carriers themselves is 1 in 4
    ☐ D in autosomal recessive disorders consanguinity is more common than in the general population
    ☐ E in autosomal dominant conditions males and females are equally affected

Genetics and Syndromes

5. **The following single gene disorders have been linked with the accompanying chromosomal locations:**

- [ ] A tuberous sclerosis 9q
- [ ] B polyposis coli 5q
- [ ] C phenylketonuria 11q
- [ ] D sickle cell disease 12q
- [ ] E cystic fibrosis 7q

6. **Prader-Willi is associated with**

- [ ] A feeding difficulties in the neonatal period
- [ ] B hyperphagia in childhood
- [ ] C blunted growth hormone response with pituitary testing
- [ ] D imperforate anus
- [ ] E cataract formation in the neonatal period

7. **Treacher Collins syndrome is associated with**

- [ ] A short stature
- [ ] B deafness
- [ ] C recurrent middle ear infections
- [ ] D azoospermia
- [ ] E delay of motor milestones

8. **The following are associated with a high arched palate:**

- [ ] A Marfan's syndrome
- [ ] B Down's syndrome
- [ ] C chronic granulomatous disease
- [ ] D homocystinuria
- [ ] E oculo-facial digital syndrome

9. The Di George sequence is associated with

- [ ] A hypocalcaemia
- [ ] B tetralogy of Fallot
- [ ] C T cell deficiency
- [ ] D short philtrum
- [ ] E choanal atresia

10. Sturge-Weber syndrome

- [ ] A is inherited as an X-linked recessive disorder
- [ ] B can be associated with epilepsy
- [ ] C is associated with B cell disorders
- [ ] D can be associated with buphthalmos
- [ ] E is associated with ventriculo-septal defects

11. Klinefelter's syndrome

- [ ] A only occurs in males
- [ ] B is associated with raised paternal age
- [ ] C is associated with short stature
- [ ] D is associated with an increased risk of breast cancer
- [ ] E related infertility is treated by testosterone replacement

ANSWERS AND TEACHING NOTES : GENETICS AND SYNDROMES

1. **B E**
   Cystic fibrosis is an autosomal recessive condition in which affected males are infertile or subfertile. There is a carrier rate of about 1 in 25 for the Western world and 70% of UK cases carry the delta 508 mutation on the short arm of chromosome 7. It is now possible to detect carriers and affected cases, the latter by both prenatal and antenatal testing. Knowing that IIa is affected suggests that both parents are carriers. Accordingly, the other children carry a 1 in 4 risk of being affected and a 2 in 3 chance of being carriers. Following from this if IIc has a 2 in 3 chance of being a carrier, his partner would have a 1 in 25 chance of being a carrier too and their offspring a further 1 in 4 risk of being affected.
   i.e. $2/3 \times 1/25 \times 1/4 = 2/300$
   i.e. a 1 in 150 chance of being affected.

2. **D E**
   Other inheritable causes of blindness are congenital cataracts, anophthalmos and retinitis pigmentosa.

3. **A E**
   X-linked recessive disorders are:
   nephrogenic diabetes insipidus
   haemophilia A and Christmas disease
   Lesch-Nyhan syndrome
   duchenne muscular dystrophy
   glucose 6 phosphate deficiency
   chronic granulomatous disease
   Hunter's disease
   Vitamin D resistant rickets is inherited in an X-linked dominant fashion.

4. **D E**
   Autosomal disorders with complete penetrance are characterised by affecting the sexes equally, with a risk of transmission of 1 in 2. An unaffected person cannot transmit the gene disorder.
   Those with autosomal recessive conditions may have normal parents who are more likely to be consanguinous. The risk of transmission to siblings however is 1 in 4.
   X-linked recessive disorders have a risk of transmission from carrier female parents to male siblings of 1 in 2. This is the same risk to daughters of carrier females being carriers themselves.

Answers and Teaching Notes: Genetics and Syndromes

5. **A B E**
   The following chromosomal locations have been linked to these diseases:
   alpha thalassaemia   16p
   beta thalassaemia   11p
   phenylketonuria   12q
   sickle cell disease   11p
   cystic fibrosis   7p
   duchenne muscular dystrophy   Xp
   tuberous sclerosis   9q
   polyposis coli   5q
   haemophilia A and B   Xq

6. **A B C**
   Prader-Willi syndrome comprises obesity, hypotonia most marked in the first year of life and small hands and feet. Feeding difficulties may occur in the neonatal period with the hyperphagic element seen in later childhood. The palpebral fissures are almond shaped and there is often a small penis and cryptorchidism.
   The IQ score is generally low, the upper range of score being about 80.
   The response of pituitary testing shows a blunted response and with the hyperinsulinism arising as a consequence of hyperphagia is thought to contribute to the obesity seen in this syndrome.

7. **B C**
   Features which are seen include antimongoloid slanting palpebral fissure, malar hypoplasia, mandibular hypoplasia, coloboma, incorrect development of pinna. Defects in the external auditory meatus are common as are conductive deafness and cleft palate. This syndrome is transmitted as an autosomal dominant condition.

8. **A D E**
   High arched palate, often seen with maxillary hypoplasia, is seen commonly in Marfan's syndrome, and less often in homocystinuria and oculo-facial digital syndrome.
   High arched palate is also seen in achondroplasia, Cockayne syndrome, Crouzon, cornelia de Lange, maternal PKU fetal effects, Rubinstein-Taybi, Treacher Collins syndrome and Turner's syndrome.
   The **skeletal abnormalities of Down's syndrome** include brachycephaly, thin cranium often with delayed fontanelle fusion, shortened hard palate, low flattened nasal bridge, irregular hypoplastic teeth, shortened metacarpals and phalanges, clinodactyly of fifth finger, pelvic hypoplasia with shallow acetabulum, atlantoaxial instability, abnormal odontoid process, 11 ribs and fusion of vertebrae.

Answers and Teaching Notes: Genetics and Syndromes

In Marfan's syndrome skeletal abnormalities include tall stature, arachnodactyly, scoliosis, kyphosis, pectus carinatum or excavatum and hemivertebrae.

Homocystinuria is associated with the features listed in Marfan's syndrome as well as osteoporosis.

The oculo-facial digital syndrome encompasses incorrect development of the hard and soft palate, anomalous and absent teeth, syndactyly, brachydactyly, clinodactyly, polydactyly, frontal bossing and hypoplasia of the mandibular ramus and zygoma.

9. A B C D E

The Di George sequence arises as a defect in the embryological development of the third and fourth pharyngeal arches affecting the formation of the thymus, parathyroid glands and the heart.

Depending on the extent of involvement there may be partial or complete absence of the thymus, parathyroids and great vessels. Hence there may be T cell deficiency, hypocalcaemia and aortic anomalies such as interrupted aortic arch, truncus arteriosus, tetralogy of Fallot. The facies tend to have a short philtrum, hypertelorism, downward slanting palpebral fissures and abnormalities of the pinna.

10. B D

Sturge Weber syndrome comprises the clinical entity of facial haemangioma often in the distribution of the trigeminal nerve with haemangiomata of arachnoid and pia mater giving rise to fitting. Paresis and decreased IQ scores may be seen. Involvement of the choroid of the eye can lead to buphthalmos when the ophthalmic distribution of the trigeminal nerve is affected.

The mode of inheritance is sporadic.

11. A D

Klinefelter's syndrome is characterised by the XXY combination of sex chromosomes and therefore can only occur in males. It is associated with raised maternal age and causes the individually affected patient to be tall and to have a low upper:lower segment ratio.

There is an increased incidence of diabetes mellitus, breast cancer and varicose veins.

Testosterone replacement therapy is recommended as it improves the development of secondary sexual characteristics. It does not affect the infertility associated with this syndrome.

STATISTICS AND EPIDEMIOLOGY

1. **In a positively skewed frequency distribution**

   - [ ] A the tail is longest going towards the origin of the axes
   - [ ] B the median is the same as the mode
   - [ ] C the median may be closer to the mode than the mean
   - [ ] D the mode is the value which occurs most frequently
   - [ ] E the median is the mid-point of the data

2. **The following tests are based on the assumption of a normal distribution:**

   - [ ] A Student's t test
   - [ ] B the chi-squared test
   - [ ] C the Mann-Whitney test
   - [ ] D the Poisson distribution
   - [ ] E confidence intervals

3. **The following are true for normal distributions:**

   - [ ] A the standard deviation is given by the mean divided by the number of components (n) of the population
   - [ ] B the square of the standard deviation of the population is the variance
   - [ ] C 66% of the observations lie within 2 standard deviations either side of the mean
   - [ ] D the geometric mean is produced by summing the logged values of a data set, dividing by n and then the mean is the resultant anti-log figure
   - [ ] E the arithmetic mean is the anti-logged figure of a skewed distribution

4. **The following statements are true:**

   - [ ] A the null hypothesis states that there is no difference between treatments or procedures being investigated
   - [ ] B the smaller the p value the less likely that the null hypothesis is correct
   - [ ] C a type 1 or alpha error occurs when the null hypothesis has been rejected incorrectly
   - [ ] D a type 2 or beta error occurs when the null hypothesis has been rejected incorrectly
   - [ ] E the power of a study is a measure of how many false positives are allowed to detect an effect at a specific size

5. The following are true about trials:

- [ ] A in an observational trial the researcher influences the events that are being studied
- [ ] B cross-sectional data look at individuals at a single time point
- [ ] C covariates do not have to be taken into account in longitudinal data sets
- [ ] D randomization is used to prevent bias
- [ ] E retrospective information used in case-control studies produces accurate data

6. The following epidemiological terms are true:

- [ ] A the prevalence of a disease is the number of persons affected by the disease divided by the number of persons in the population at one point or period in time
- [ ] B the incidence rate is the number of new cases of disease in a given time period divided by the total person-time of observation during that time
- [ ] C the cumulative incidence is the total number of cases of the disease in a given time period divided by the number of people at the beginning of the time period
- [ ] D the sensitivity of a test is given by the ratio of the number of actual positive values divided by the total of actual positives and false negatives
- [ ] E the specificity of a test relates to the ratio of false positive values compared with the total of false positive values and true negative values

7. The following statements are true:

- [ ] A the perinatal mortality rate is the total number of stillbirths and early neonatal deaths per year per 1000 live births
- [ ] B the early neonatal death rate is the number of deaths within 30 days of life per 1000 live births
- [ ] C the perinatal mortality figures are increased above the maternal age of 35 years and below the age of 20 years
- [ ] D 80% of all neonatal deaths occur in the first week of life
- [ ] E cardiovascular anomalies account for 35–40% of all neonatal deaths

Statistics and Epidemiology

8. **The following question relates to the causes of death in the United Kingdom:**

   - [ ] A in the first year of life the commonest cause is accidents
   - [ ] B between the ages of 1 to 4 years the second commonest cause is neoplasia
   - [ ] C from the ages of 5 to 9 years the commonest cause is infection
   - [ ] D from 10 to 14 years infections are the fourth commonest cause
   - [ ] E sixteen is the average number of deaths per year in the age range 0–14 years per million children

9. **The following relate to measures of risk of being affected by a disease after exposure compared with a non-exposed population:**

   - [ ] A the absolute risk of a condition is the rate of occurrence
   - [ ] B the relative risk is given as the incidence among the affected people and the incidence in the non-exposed divided by the incidence in the non-exposed
   - [ ] C the attributable risk is the difference between the rate of incidence in the exposed from the incidence in the non-exposed
   - [ ] D the population attributable risk is the sum of the prevalence of the attributable risk and the prevalence of the risk factor in the population
   - [ ] E the population attributable risk fraction is given by the population attributable risk being divided by the incidence in the whole population (i.e. exposed and non-exposed)

10. **To look at the features of a new test X compared with the 'standard reference test'**

	STANDARD TEST	
	Positive	Negative
TEST X		
Positive	TRUE + (A)	FALSE + (B)
Negative	FALSE –ve (C)	TRUE –ve (D)
	Total with disease (A + C)	Total without disease (B + D)

    - [ ] A the sensitivity of the test $X = A / A + C$
    - [ ] B the specificity of test $X = D / B + C$
    - [ ] C the predictive value of a positive test $= A / A + B$
    - [ ] D the predictive value of a negative test $= B / C + D$
    - [ ] E the number of test negatives for test $X = C + B$

ANSWERS AND TEACHING NOTES : STATISTICS AND EPIDEMIOLOGY

1. **D E**
   The tail is longer on the right rather than towards the origin of the axes. In a positively skewed distribution the mean is greater than the median which is greater than the mode. The reverse holds true for a negatively skewed distribution.
   The median is the middle value of a set of observations which have been ranked in order. The mode is the value which occurs most frequently. The mean is given by the sum of all the values divided by the number of values present in the data set.

2. **A E**
   Tests which rely on a parametric that is a normal distribution include Student's t test and confidence intervals.

3. **B D**
   The standard deviation of a normally distributed data set is calculated by first obtaining the figure for the difference between each of the points of data from the mean of the data set, squaring this figure and adding together the squared figures then dividing this resultant sum by n less 1.
   95% of observations lie within 2 standard deviations of the mean, 68% lie within 1 standard deviation and 99.7% within 3 standard deviations.
   The geometric mean is used in skewed data whereas the arithmetric mean is the figure produced by summing the values of the data set and dividing by n.

4. **A B C E**
   The null hypothesis considers that there is no difference between whatever is being compared hence the larger p becomes (i.e. the greater the likelihood that what was seen was due to chance) the closer the null hypothesis is to being confirmed.
   It is always important to remember that a statistically significant result does not necessarily have clinical significance.
   The type 2 or beta error occurs when the null hypothesis has been accepted incorrectly.
   The power of a study may be set so as to accept 5% false positives which will then allow a size to observe this effect to be calculated.

5. **B D**
   An observational trial is one in which the observer remains independent of the study and does not influence the events being measured or monitored. An experimental study is the opposite in that the researcher is directly altering one or more of the components of the study to ascertain an effect.

Answers and Teaching Notes: Statistics and Epidemiology

Cross-sectional studies are concerned with looking at data at one single point in time – a 'snap-shot' as opposed to longitudinal data which looks at data in a sequence of time.

Covariates are data such as age or height or other biological data which might have an influence on the results of the study.

In comparative studies looking at groups of observations, these observations are compared in all aspects other than that being compared! The use of randomisation helps to remove the bias by allowing treatments between the groups which do not differ in any systematic way. Hence random selection removes unconscious or willing error produced by the observer in comparing the treatments.

Retrospective studies using matched controls with cases are often biased as people affected by an illness may have considered possible aetiological factors compared with healthy individuals who have not had reason to speculate in this fashion.

6. **A B D**

The cumulative incidence is the number of new cases of disease in a given period of time divided by the number of people at the beginning of the time period.

The specificity is the ratio of the number of true negatives to the total of false positives and true negatives.

7. **C D E**

The perinatal mortality rate is the number of stillbirths and early neonatal deaths occurring per year per 1000 *total births*.

The majority of neonatal deaths occur early in life. Early neonatal deaths comprise 46% of infant deaths and 23% of all childhood deaths.

Congenital abnormalities such as cardiovascular anomalies account for 35–40% of causes of neonatal deaths whereas central nervous system disorders and respiratory disorders comprise 13–15% of these deaths.

8. **D**

In the first year of life the **causes of death** are given in order of occurrence as:
    congenital abnormalities
    prematurity
    birth asphyxia/trauma
    sudden infant cot death syndrome
    infections
    accidents
    central nervous system disorders.

Between 1 to 4 years the causes of death are given in order of occurrence as:
   congenital abnormalities
   accidents
   infections
   neoplasia
   central nervous system disorders.
Between 5 to 9 years the causes of death are given in order of occurrence as:
   accidents
   neoplasia
   congenital abnormalities
   infections.
Between 10 to 14 years the causes of death are:
   accidents
   neoplasia
   central nervous system disorders.
Overall the mortality rate for children aged from birth to 14 years is 164 per million children per year.

9. **A C E**
The relative risk is the ratio of the exposed divided by the incidence of the same disease in the non-exposed.
The population attributable risk is the PRODUCT of the attributable risk and the prevalence of the risk factor in the population
Odds ratios are also given. This is the ratio of the probability of an episode/occurrence divided by 1- the probability of the episode/occurrence and approximates to the relative risk when the incidence/prevalence of the disease is low.

10. **A B**
The specificity of test X = D / B and D, the predictive value of a negative test = D / C and D. The number of test negatives for test X = C and D, the number of test postives for test X being A + B.
The test bias is given as the ratio of the test positives divided by the number of true (i.e. standard) positives = A + B / A + C.

IMMUNISATION

1. **The following vaccines can be given to HIV positive individuals:**

   - A yellow fever
   - B whooping cough
   - C rubella
   - D live polio vaccine
   - E BCG

2. **The following are contraindications to immunisation:**

   - A a family history of convulsions
   - B previous history of measles
   - C prematurity
   - D cerebral palsy
   - E a family history of adverse reactions following immunisation

3. **The following statements about BCG are true:**

   - A neonates who have been in contact with tuberculosis should be given BCG
   - B contacts of sputum positive patients may show a negative tuberculin test because they are in the early stages of infection
   - C veterinary staff who deal with simians are at higher risk
   - D if BCG is given to infants, polio vaccine should be delayed for 3 months
   - E no other immunisation should be given in the same arm as the BCG vaccination for 2 weeks

4. **The reaction to tuberculin may be suppressed by the following factors:**

   - A sarcoidosis
   - B glandular fever
   - C live viral vaccines
   - D upper respiratory tract infection
   - E Hodgkin's disease

5. The following are true about the Heaf test:

- [ ] A grade 3 Heaf reaction describes a uniform circle of induration 5–10 mm width at each needle site
- [ ] B a subject with a grade 1 Heaf reaction who gives a history of previous BCG but who does not have a characteristic scar should be re-immunised
- [ ] C subjects previously immunised with BCG who show a grade 4 reaction should be reassured
- [ ] D grade 1 reaction consists of discrete indurations at four or more needle sites
- [ ] E the Heaf test can be read accurately 10 days after having been given

6. Specific immunoglobulin is available for

- [ ] A tetanus
- [ ] B measles
- [ ] C mumps
- [ ] D rabies
- [ ] E hepatitis B

7. Yellow fever

- [ ] A vaccine is an inactivated freeze-dried preparation of yellow fever virus
- [ ] B vaccine can be given within 24 hours of being reconstituted
- [ ] C immunity persists for at least 10 years
- [ ] D vaccine can be given safely to pregnant women
- [ ] E encephalitis can occur rarely in infants following immunisation and resolves in the majority without sequelae

8. Anaphylaxis following immunisation

- [ ] A is indicated by a strong central pulse
- [ ] B may be heralded by feelings of retrosternal tightness
- [ ] C may present with apnoea, pallor and limpness
- [ ] D should be treated with 1/1000 strength adrenaline given by the deep intramuscular route in the absence of an adequate cardiac output
- [ ] E adrenaline doses may be repeated up to a maximum of three times

ANSWERS AND TEACHING NOTES : IMMUNISATION

1. **B C D**
   Yellow fever and BCG are not recommended to be given to HIV positive individuals. Live vaccines such as measles, mumps, rubella and polio may be given. Live polio is excreted in the stool for longer periods than in unaffected people. Inactivated vaccines which may be given include whooping cough, diphtheria, tetanus, inactivated polio, cholera, hepatitis B, typhoid and Hib.

2. **ALL FALSE**
   A family history of adverse reactions or of convulsions is not a contraindication to immunisation. Previous infection with whooping cough, mumps, rubella or measles similarly does not prevent immunisation. Immunisation should not be postponed in the case of prematurity. Stable neurological disorders such as cerebral palsy are not a contraindication to immunisation.

3. **B**
   Groups at higher risk of infection include health service staff, veterinary staff and other staff who handle animal species known to be susceptible to tuberculosis, unimmunised contacts of cases known to be suffering from open pulmonary tuberculosis, immigrants from countries with a high prevalence of the disease and those intending to stay in Asia, Africa and the Southern/Central Americas.

   Neonates who are contacts should receive prophylactic isoniazid treatment and after 3–6 weeks should be re-tested with the tuberculin test. If positive, antibiotic treatment is continued. If the tuberculin test is negative, BCG is given as long as they are not in contact with an infective tuberculosis contact.

   BCG should not be given to subjects on steroid or immunosuppressive therapy, receiving radiotherapy, suffering from a disorder of the reticulo-endothelial system such as lymphoma, leukaemia or Hodgkin's disease, in immunologically disturbed conditions such as hypogammaglobulinaemia, HIV positive individuals, those who are pregnant, are pyrexial or have extensive generalised skin disease.

   BCG should be separated from other vaccines by an interval of three weeks and the same arm not used for a period of three months as there is a risk of regional lymphadenitis developing.

   In infants, oral polio replicates in the intestine inducing local immunity as well as causing the development of serum antibodies.

4. **A B C D E**
   Corticosteroid therapy, viral infections in general, immunosuppressive disorders including HIV also suppress the tuberculin response.

   Other variables such as skin thickness and reactivity may vary in different parts of the body hence the recommended site on the flexor surface of the left forearm at the junction of the lower two-thirds with the upper third.

With increasing age there is a diminished response to tuberculin testing.

5. **A B D E**

The **Heaf test** is performed by using tuberculin 100,000 units/ml solution to cover an area on the flexor surface of the left forearm slightly greater than the head of the Heaf gun. This gun has six needles which inject to a preset depth and introduce the tuberculin intradermally. Residual tuberculin solution is wiped off the skin and the site is observed to ensure that there are six discrete puncture marks.

The reaction is read 3–10 days following administration.

Grade 0	No induration
Grade 1	Discrete induration at four or more puncture marks
Grade 2	A circle of induration formed by coalescing of reaction around each needle site, but with a clear area within the circle of the puncture marks
Grade 3	A completely filled circle of induration, 5–10 mm in diameter
Grade 4	The circle of induration is greater than 10 mm in diameter

Subjects with grade 0 and 1 reactions are said to have a negative result and should be offered BCG immunisation.

Grade 2 reactors are individuals who demonstrate a hypersensitivity to tuberculin protein and so should not be given BCG.

Grade 3 and grade 4 subjects should be referred for further investigation, including those people previously immunised with BCG.

6. **A D E**

Specific immunoglobulins exist for rabies, hepatitis B, tetanus and varicella/zoster.

Rabies

Rabies specific immunoglobulin is given to the unimmunised subject who has been biten by a rabid animal. The subject should be immunised with the human diploid cell rabies vaccine by deep subcutaneous or intramuscular injection on the day of the bite, then at day 3, 7, 14, 30 and 90 following the day of the bite. Around the site of the entry wound which must have been thoroughly cleaned, rabies specific immunoglobulin 10 iu/kg body weight is infiltrated and a further 10 iu/kg body weight is given in a different site to where the vaccine is administered.

Answers and Teaching Notes: Immunisation

Hepatitis B (HBIG)
HBIG is used to produce immediate protection and is given with the vaccine at a different site to the vaccination. In the neonate, passive and active immunisation must be given within 48 hours of birth. This should be performed on all babies whose mothers have been infected with hepatitis B including those who are only HBsAg positive.

Tetanus
Immunoglobulin is recommended to be given to subjects who last received tetanus vaccination more than 10 years ago. It is also recommended to subjects who are not immunised or who are unclear of their vaccination status.

Varicella/Zoster (VZIG)
VZIG is recommended for
1. neonates whose mothers had developed chickenpox 7 days to 1 month prior to delivery, to neonates who have been in contact with zoster/chickenpox and those whose mothers do not have a history of chickenpox exposure or who have no antibody to chickenpox on testing
2. immunosuppressed or immunocompromised subjects
3. all bone marrow recipients irrespective of past varicella/zoster status
4. pregnant women with undetectable antibody levels to chickenpox
5. HIV positive individuals with symptoms who are negative for varicella/zoster antibody.

Human normal immunoglobulin (HNIG), prepared from pooled antibody, is used for prophylaxis of measles and hepatitis A. It is given by deep intramuscular injection; its efficacy depends on the current prevalence of those viruses in the population from which the antibody has been collected.

HNIG is used in immunosuppressed or immunocompromised subjects who have been exposed to measles and offers short term protection against hepatitis A. It is also recommended for travellers to regions of endemic hepatitis A and in the control of outbreaks of infection. HNIG is not recommended to prevent infection with rubella or mumps.

7. **C E**
Yellow fever vaccine is a live attenuated vaccine and should be given within an hour of reconstitution, by the deep subcutaneous route.
Immunity lasts for at least 10 years but the vaccine cannot be given to pregnant women. Encephalitis has been seen in infants and in the majority of these cases has resolved without sequelae.

Answers and Teaching Notes: Immunisation

Contraindications to its administration include: febrile illness, steroid therapy, immunosuppressive treatment, immunodeficiency syndromes, reticuloendothelial disorders, hypersensitivity reactions to polymixin/neomycin, anaphylactic reactions to egg, HIV positive status.

Generally infants under the age of 9 months are vaccinated if the risk of yellow fever is unavoidable.

8. **B C D E**

Anaphylaxis is a rare occurence, 118 cases being reported in the period 1978–1989 in the UK during which time 25 million childhood immunisation were performed.

The differential diagnoses are fits and faints. Young children uncommonly faint and the sudden loss of consciousness should be managed as a case of anaphylaxis in the absence of an adequate cardiac output which is maintained in a fit or a faint.

Symptoms commonest in childhood are pallor, apnoea and limpness. Upper airway obstruction due to angio-oedema causes stridor and hoarseness. Lower airway obstruction gives rise to retrosternal tightness and wheeze. There may be a marked tachycardia, or bradycardia. A key feature which is seen is hypotension. Dermatological manifestations include urticaria and weals.

The subject should be placed in the left lateral position. The airway should be maintained and the resuscitator should shout for help. Then 1/1000 adrenaline is given by deep intramuscular injection in the presence of poor cardiac output whilst cardiopulmonary resuscitation is carried out. If there is no improvement after 10 minutes a further dose of adrenaline may be given, which may be repeated after a further 10 minutes.

High flow oxygen should be given throughout with repeated reassessment of the airway and adequate cardiopulmonary resuscitation being effected.

All subjects who have had an anaphylactic reaction must be admitted for observation and notification of the reaction must be made to the Committee on Safety of Medicines.

SURGERY

1. **In tracheo-oesophageal fistula**

   ☐ A the incidence is 1 in 1000
   ☐ B gas is never present in the bowel
   ☐ C primary end-to-end anastomosis can be formed where there is a narrow gap between the oesophageal ends
   ☐ D colonic implantation may be necessary
   ☐ E the H-type is the commonest form

2. **Exomphalos**

   ☐ A has an incidence of 1 in 5000
   ☐ B is associated with major abnormalities in 10% of cases
   ☐ C is associated with Beckwith-Wiedemann syndrome
   ☐ D can lead to respiratory distress when primary reduction and closure is carried out
   ☐ E is a sac made of the amniotic membrane and peritoneum

3. **Urethral valves**

   ☐ A are associated most often with involvement of the anterior valves
   ☐ B present in late childhood with incontinence
   ☐ C present with distended bladder
   ☐ D can be diagnosed in utero
   ☐ E commonly cause renal aplasia

4. **The following statements about testes are true:**

   ☐ A epididymo-orchitis requires surgical exploration
   ☐ B a retractile testis requires surgical fixation
   ☐ C an ectopic testis requires surgical fixation
   ☐ D torsion of the testis occurs most commonly between the ages of 3 and 5 years
   ☐ E the hydatid of Morgani is the most common embryological remnant to undergo torsion

5. Pyloric stenosis

- [ ] A gives rise to bile stained vomit
- [ ] B is associated with metabolic acidosis
- [ ] C needs a gallium scan to confirm the diagnosis
- [ ] D resolves with medical treatment
- [ ] E occurs more often in females

ANSWERS AND TEACHING NOTES : SURGERY

1. **C D**
   The incidence of this condition is 1 in 3500, the commonest form being a blind ending oesophagus with the trachea joining the lower bud from the stomach near the carina. Gas is present in the bowel as there has to be a communication between the trachea and the remainder of the bowel. In small distances between the ends of the oesophagus a direct anastomosis can be formed.
   With large gaps between the ends of the oesophageal ends, interposition of colonic tissue may be used to fashion a new conduit. The H-type of tracheo-oesophageal fistula only accounts for 4% of cases, presenting often due to aspiration of food via the fistula to cause recurrent chest infections.

2. **A C D**
   The incidence of associated abnormalities is about 40%, with syndromes such as Beckwith-Wiedemann syndrome, Edward's syndrome and Patau's syndrome. Respiratory distress may occur secondary to compression of the diaphragm. An omphalocoele is the sac of fused amniotic membrane and peritoneum. An exomphalos is due to herniation into the umbilical cord of gut contents. This may include viscera such as liver, spleen and bowel.

3. **B C D**
   The posterior urethal valves are mucosal folds attached by the verumontanum. These come together when micturition is initiated.
   Ultrasound scan can make the diagnosis in utero and it presents in the neonatal period with a distended bladder and dilation of the posterior portion of the urethra. Urine may be passed in dribbling fashion or there may be complete retention.
   Bladder hypertrophy may occur but the kidneys are usually unaffected. Later in childhood the presentation may be with incontinence with persistent passage of urine.

4. **C E**
   Epididymo-orchitis requires treatment with antibiotics. If there is any doubt about the diagnosis then surgical exploration is required. A retractile testis occurs due to the cremasteric reflex which draws the testis into the superficial inguinal pouch. The retractile testis can be brought down by manipulation into the scrotum and does not require surgical fixation as descent will occur with time.
   Malignancy occurs in 0.002% of adult males with over 12% of cases occurring in undescended testes, an increased incidence of 40%.
   Some of the embryological remnants such as the hydatid of Morgani, are Mullerian duct remnants. The Wolffian tubercle gives rise to the appendix, epididymis and the vas aberrans of Haller.

Torsion of the testis occurs most often in the neonatal period or in puberty. The other testis must be fixed at the time of exploration.

5. **ALL FALSE**

The obstruction in pyloric stenosis is proximal to the sphincter of Oddi, hence the vomitus is not bile stained.

With persistent vomiting metabolic alkalosis results from loss of hydrochloric acid. Hypokalaemia can result as the renal compensation to preserve sodium gives rise to increased potassium loss in the urine.

The diagnosis can be made by a test feed – an ultrasound or barium meal will comfirm the gastric outlet obstruction.

Pyloric stenosis requires a pyloromyotomy, Ramstedt's operation.

It has a polygenic mode of inheritance and occurs more commonly in males.

PSYCHIATRY/PSYCHO-SOCIAL PAEDIATRICS

1. **Sleep problems in children**

   - A are commonest in the 5–8 age group
   - B should be treated with trimeprazine
   - C require benzodiazepines to control the situation
   - D can be helped by short term use of chloral hydrate
   - E in the form of nightmares are often related to a frightening experience

2. **Schizophrenia**

   - A does not occur in prepubertal children
   - B is associated with auditory hallucinations that may respond to ear plugs
   - C is associated with visual hallucinations that may respond to distorting glasses
   - D associated hallucinations do not occur without concurrent psychosis
   - E has no available medication in childhood

3. **Extrapyramidal side-effects of neuroleptics include**

   - A neuroleptic malignant syndrome occuring only in the first 6 hours of therapy
   - B oculogyric crises
   - C akinesia
   - D tardive dystonia
   - E gynaecomastia

4. **Bipolar illness in childhood**

   - A is autosomal recessively inherited
   - B has onset usually by 8 years of age
   - C is usually treated with lithium
   - D is associated with increased toxicity to therapy in hot weather
   - E can be treated with carbamazepine

5. Incontinence

- [ ] A in the form of enuresis must be fully investigated by 3 years of age
- [ ] B in the form of encopresis must be fully investigated by 3 years of age
- [ ] C is often associated with constipation
- [ ] D tends to occur in families
- [ ] E of urine can be managed with amitriptyline

6. In epilepsy

- [ ] A behavioural problems are only drug related
- [ ] B carbamazepine is associated with behavioural problems at low therapeutic levels
- [ ] C changing to vigabactrin markedly improves difficult distressed children
- [ ] D treatment with benzodiazepines can interfere with accurate neuropsychology assessments
- [ ] E behavioural problems can be well controlled with dexamphetamine

7. In the courts

- [ ] A a child under 10 years cannot be found guilty of a crime
- [ ] B a child can be found guilty of homicide at any age
- [ ] C a child should not be prosecuted for a crime between the ages of 9 and 16
- [ ] D a child under 14 years should only present for care proceedings
- [ ] E there are increasing numbers of boys and girls presenting

8. Anorexia nervosa

- [ ] A tends to occur before 12 years of age
- [ ] B does not occur in boys
- [ ] C is most common in social classes I and II
- [ ] D is associated with an increased incidence of eating disorders in relatives
- [ ] E consists of a disturbance of body image

Psychiatry/Psycho-Social Paediatrics

9. Associated factors in anorexia nervosa include

- [ ] A below average intelligence
- [ ] B low exercise rate
- [ ] C 5–10% mortality
- [ ] D cardiac arrhythmias
- [ ] E electrolyte disturbance

10. Child abuse

- [ ] A only occurs in social class V
- [ ] B is more common in single parent families
- [ ] C is more common in high unemployment areas
- [ ] D is only carried out by the parents
- [ ] E may often have occurred to the offender in the past

11. Recognised clinical features of childhood autism include:

- [ ] A echolalia
- [ ] B specific preoccupations with unusual objects
- [ ] C 90% have an intelligence quotient above 100
- [ ] D symptoms present after 5 years
- [ ] E 15% develop fits as teenagers

12. The differential diagnoses of hypomanic/manic episodes include

- [ ] A encephalitis
- [ ] B glioma
- [ ] C antituberculous drugs
- [ ] D hyperthyroidism
- [ ] E repeated fitting

ANSWERS AND TEACHING NOTES :
PSYCHIATRY/PSYCHO-SOCIAL PAEDIATRICS

1. **D E**
   Sleep problems are most common in the toddler years when there is difficulty in settling, fear of intruders and early morning rising. Drug treatment should be strictly avoided, especially benzodiazepines which may lead to worse behavioural problems. In desperate situations with exhausted parents a small dose of chloral hydrate can occasionally be tried. Children usually respond far better to behavioural therapy. Similarly nightmares can be traced back to a frightening experience in the majority of situations and drug treatment should be avoided if possible.

2. **B C**
   Adult type schizophrenia although rare pre-pubertally, does occur in childhood. It is most frequently found in adolescents. Management must be in a specialist unit. Some simple measures can help control symptoms, for example putting an ear plug in the most affected side for auditory hallucinations and using distorting glasses for visual hallucinations. These problems can be most disabling as they can occur with or without psychosis. Drug treatment consists of neuroleptics as with adults and results are very variable, with similar problems of side effects also occurring in all age groups.

3. **B C D**
   Neuroleptics (for example chlorpromazine, thioridazine and haloperidol) used in the treatment of schizophrenia have many severe extrapyramidal side-effects. Acute dystonias such as oculogyric crises may occur at any time in the first week of starting treatment. Akathesia (an unpleasant restless agitation) may occur at any time from within hours to two months after the start of treatment and Parkinsonian symptoms (rigidity, tremor and akinesis) may occur within the first month of starting treatment. Tardive dyskinesia and tardive akathesia may occur several months after neuroleptic therapy, whilst tardive dystonia may occur from a few days to after a decade of therapy. Neuroleptic malignant syndrome can occur at any time. Symptoms may improve with procylidine in an emergency.

   Non-extrapyramidal symptoms include galactorrhoea, gynaecomastia, weight gain and jaundice.

4. **C D E**
   Bipolar manic/depressive disorder in childhood is a problem of the teenage years and is almost never seen before this age. The form of inheritance, if it exists, is not known. Treatment is with lithium carbonate, levels being carefully monitored to avoid toxicity consisting of diarrhoea, vomiting, tremor, ataxia, dysarthria, muscle weakness, cardiac arrythmias and coma. Thyroid dysfunction may also occur and a degree of nephrotoxicity has caused concern.

Answers and Teaching Notes: Psychiatry/Psycho-Social Paediatrics

An alternative therapy in non-responsive cases is carbamazepine, it may even be preferable in children who rapidly change in their manic/depressive cycles.

5. **C D E**
   Enuresis and encopresis can lead to great distress to the child and family. Generally for developmental reasons encopresis is investigated from 4 years of age, with initial investigation into clinical causes, for example constipation, and concentration on behavioural therapy. There are frequently major underlying psychological problems in children with soiling. Nocturnal enuresis is investigated from around 5 years, ensuring no underlying urodynamic problems exist and then progressing into behavioural therapy. Examples of such therapy may be the 'bell and pad' and star charts. Rarely is it necessary to resort to amitryptiline or imipramine, but these should be avoided if possible.

6. **D E**
   Epilepsy is well known to be associated with major behavioural problems in children, this is believed to be related to the underlying condition as well as the medication. Carbamazepine can make behaviour worse (when well into the therapeutic range), as can benzodiazepines, occasionally leading to pseudodementia, making children on longterm therapy very difficult to assess. Vigabactrin is also associated with major behavioural problems to the point of causing psychosis in a few cases. Where it is absolutely necessary therapy with dexamphetamine can improve the situation and is believed to raise the seizure threshold.

7. **B D E**
   In the United Kingdom a child under 10 years cannot be found guilty of a crime unless it is murder and should not be prosecuted for a crime between 10–14 years of age. So children under 14 years of age should only present to court for care proceedings. The primary role of supervision orders is to advise, assist and befriend offenders and not to protect the public, although repeated offenders will be returned to court for the situation to be reviewed.

   There are increasing numbers of both boys and girls now presenting, although the majority are male and they often continue to commit crimes.

8. **C D E**
   Anorexia nervosa is a condition affecting girls, it rarely occurs in boys. It mainly affects girls in two age peaks of 14.5 and 18 years. The condition is most common in social classes I and II and occasionally in certain ethnic groups, especially where avoidance of puberty and consequent responsibilities are desired.

   There is an increased incidence of eating disorders in relatives.

Answers and Teaching Notes: Psychiatry/Psycho-Social Paediatrics

Important diagnostic factors include persistent fear of becoming obese, disturbance of body image, weight loss of at least 25% of natural body weight, refusal to maintain weight and absence of known physical disease which could be responsible for weight loss.

9. **C D E**
Adolescents with anorexia nervosa tend to be above average intelligence, often very obsessional, manipulative and hard working. They will carefully measure out foods, count calories and have a very high exercise rate. The condition carries a 5–10% mortality, death usually being related to severe emaciation with cardiac arrthymias secondary to electrolyte imbalance. This occurs with poor dietary input and high incidence of diuretic/laxative abuse and induced emesis. Poor diet can also lead to bone marrow impairment with associated leucopenia and anaemia. Affected patients are notoriously resistant to treatment.

10. **B C E**
Child abuse has always existed but only recently been brought to medical and public awareness. It is recognised in several different forms:
   – physical abuse
   – neglect
   – sexual abuse
   – Munchausen by proxy.

It is more common in highly stressed families and thus can occur in any social class. But single parent families and unemployment will place a tremendous burden on the family. Abuse is not restricted to the parents alone but may be carried out by anyone able to gain access to the child. Munchausen by proxy is more commonly carried out by mothers and sexual abuse more often by men.

Unfortunately children who have been abused in whatever form do have an increased risk of going on to abuse their own children.

11. **A B E**
Children with autism have impaired social relationships, fail to co-operate in play and reject reciprocal play. There is commonly a lack of eye-to-eye gaze and facial expression with a paucity of body language and empathy.

Language may be delayed in development with echolalia an important feature.

Activities are limited with a preoccupation for unusual objects and stereotypical patterns of behaviour. Seemingly trivial alterations in the routine environment may cause distress.

In most cases symptoms present before 30 months, with 75% of children having intelligence quotients in the retarded range.

Answers and Teaching Notes: Psychiatry/Psycho-Social Paediatrics

12. A B C D E
Infections such as encephalitis, endocrine disorders eg. hyperthyroidism, central nervous disorders eg. repeated fitting, head injury, strokes, malignancies such as glioma and meningioma, drugs such as steroids and antituberculous medication and substance abuse with alcohol and amphetamines.

Causes for hypomanic/manic episodes include:
Encephalitis
Endocrine disorders eg. hyperthyroidism
Central nervous disorders
  eg. fitting
      head injury
      strokes
      malignancies
      meningiomas
Drugs eg. steroids
      anti-TB treatment
Substance abuse with alcohol and amphetamines.

ACCIDENT AND EMERGENCY

1. **A 2-year-old boy is brought to the Accident and Emergency department with a history of 'near drowning'**

   - [ ] A drowning is the second commonest cause of accidental death in children in the United Kingdom
   - [ ] B ventricular fibrillation may be resistant at temperatures below normal body temperature
   - [ ] C resuscitation should be continued until the core body temperature exceeds 32 degrees Centigrade, when the clincal status must be reassessed
   - [ ] D rewarming may lead to hypovolaemia
   - [ ] E salt water drowning carries a worse prognosis

2. **The following are true:**

   - [ ] A adrenaline may be given via the endotracheal tube in resuscitation
   - [ ] B adrenaline and atropine may be given via the same intravenous route without an intervening flush
   - [ ] C adrenaline and sodium bicarbonate may be administered through the same intravenous route without an intervening flush
   - [ ] D adrenaline may be given via an intra-osseous needle
   - [ ] E the initial endotracheal dose of adrenaline in the paediatric resuscitation is twice the intravenous dose

3. **Supraventricular tachycardia**

   - [ ] A in a shocked patient requires the administration of adenosine 50 µg/kg
   - [ ] B can occur with Wolff-Parkinson-White syndrome
   - [ ] C in the stable child invariably responds to bilateral carotid sinus massage
   - [ ] D is seen in association with Ebstein's anomaly
   - [ ] E must be treated with a combination of propranolol and digoxin

4. **The following situations are absolute contraindications to organ donation:**

   - [ ] A where there are neoplasms limited to the central nervous system
   - [ ] B where the donor has hepatitis e antigen positive serology
   - [ ] C bacteriuria in the donor excludes renal transplantation
   - [ ] D partially treated tuberculosis in donor
   - [ ] E acute tubular necrosis excludes renal transplantation

5. In children

- [ ] A ventricular fibrillation secondary to coronary arterial occlusion due to atheroma is the commonest cause of death
- [ ] B the resuscitation of hypothermic children should cease after 20 minutes provided full discussion with the parents has occured
- [ ] C in resuscitation the airway must be maintained as a first priority
- [ ] D peripheral vascular access should be sought for no longer than 20 minutes before attempting central access
- [ ] E the approximate formula for the internal diameter in millimetres for an endotracheal tube for a child aged more than 1 year is age/4 + 12

ANSWERS AND TEACHING NOTES : ACCIDENT AND EMERGENCY

1. **B C D**
   Drowning is the third commonest cause of death due to accidents, being exceeded by road traffic accidents and burns.
   Cardiac arrhythmias commonly occur and may be resistant at lower temperatures.
   Children cannot be assessed accurately at these low core body temperatures and must be warmed to above 32 degrees before reliable examination may be performed.
   On rewarming vasodilation gives rise to hypovolaemia, hence fluid replacement must be anticipated.
   There is no difference in mortality rates between fresh water and salt water drowning.

2. **A B D**
   Adrenaline, lignocaine and naloxone may all be given via the endotracheal tube. A flush should be administered to aid delivery of drugs used in resuscitation. However adrenaline and bicarbonate are incompatible in the same intravenous line. Adrenaline with lignocaine, atropine, etc may be given via the intra-osseus needle.
   The initial endotracheal dose of adrenaline is 100 micrograms per kilogram of body weight whereas the intravenous dosage is 10 micrograms per kilogram.

3. **B D**
   A child who is shocked due to a supraventricular tachycardia should, after attention to Airway, Breathing and Circulation, be shocked with synchronised DC current. The initial dose should be 0.5 J/kg. Failing a response to this dose, 1 J/kg and then if no change, 2 J/kg should be given.
   Wolf-Parkinson-White syndrome is associated with re-entry circuits to the atria causing sporadic runs of supraventricular tachycardia. Ebstein's anomaly with atrialization of the right ventricle is associated with re-entry pathways.
   In the stable child, a cold flannel or putting the child's head face first into a bucket of cold water may stimulate the diving reflex to cease the supraventricular tachycardia. Unilateral carotid sinus massage may have a similar effect. Note: bilateral carotid sinus massage may stop blood flow to the brain and therefore is not recommended.
   Propranolol and digoxin may be a fatal combination and therefore is not recommended.

4. **B D**
   Absolute contraindications to organ donation are:
   The expressed wish of the donor not to donate organs
   The possibility of hepatitis B infectivity

The presence of HIV infection
Tumours being present in the donor apart from those involving the central nervous system only, or in situ or localised to the skin.

It should be noted that age is not an absolute contraindication for donating or receiving organs and that patients who have received kidneys which had bacteriuria in the donor must have a course of antibiotic treatment after transplantation.

5. C

Ventricular fibrillation secondary to coronary occlusion due to atheroma is uncommon in childhood!

Hypothermia requires prolonged cardiopulmonary resuscitation until the core temperature is above 32 degrees Centigrade.

In the process of resuscitation, the order of priory is airway, (with cervical neck stabilisation if there has been any trauma), breathing and then the circulation.

Two attempts at securing peripheral vascular access before the use of an intra-osseous needle are generally recommended. Central access should only be attempted by physicians trained and familiar with obtaining this mode of access.

A rough guide to the required size of endotracheal tube in millimetres is given by the formula age/4 + 4 for a child over the age of 1 year. A size below and above should be kept in close proximity. If there is any suspicion that the size required may be smaller, such as in the child with croup (a smaller tube may be necessary owing to the presence of inflammation and oedema), a full range of endotracheal tubes must be available from the size above the predicted size downwards.

PRACTICE EXAM

This practice examination consists of 60 paediatric questions, unlike the official examination which contains 30 paediatric questions and 30 general medicine questions.

Time allowed 2½ hours. Mark your answers with a tick (True) or a cross (False) in the box provided. Leave the box empty for "Don't know".

1. **In the anatomy of the kidney**

   ☐ A the cortex is found within the medulla
   ☐ B the renal pyramids lie within the cortex
   ☐ C the renal pelvis is lined by squamous epithelium
   ☐ D the glomeruli proximal tubules and distal tubules are situated within the cortex
   ☐ E the loops of Henlé and the collecting ducts extend down through the medulla

2. **Antidiuretic hormone**

   ☐ A is released secondary to thirst, detected by the lateral preoptic receptors
   ☐ B is primarily synthesised in the supraoptic nucleus of the hypothalamus
   ☐ C is referred to as 8-lysine vasopressin in humans
   ☐ D after synthesis is transported to the neurohypophysis in the anterior pituitary
   ☐ E plasma half-life is about one hour

3. **The following statements are true:**

   ☐ A the plasma ionised calcium level is usually about 2.5 mmol/l
   ☐ B all plasma calcium is filtered by the kidney
   ☐ C calcium is reabsorbed from the descending loop of Henlé
   ☐ D frusemide inhibits calcium reabsorption
   ☐ E calcium is reabsorbed from each part of the nephron

4. **Serum complement 3 levels are**

   ☐ A reduced in membranous glomerulonephritis
   ☐ B raised in Goodpasture's disease
   ☐ C normal in membranoproliferative glomerulonephritis
   ☐ D reduced in Henoch-Schonlein purpura
   ☐ E normal in acute poststreptococcal glomerulonephritis

5. Infantile polycystic disease

- [ ] A often involves the liver and kidney
- [ ] B has many cysts within the renal cortex only
- [ ] C cysts are dilatations of the collecting ducts
- [ ] D may present in a Potter syndrome pattern
- [ ] E occasionally presents as nephrogenic diabetes insipidus

6. Vertical transmission of HIV

- [ ] A occurs only before birth
- [ ] B is more likely to occur in infected mothers with low CD4 counts
- [ ] C is less likely to occur if infected infants deliver prematurely to infected mothers
- [ ] D has an increased incidence in infants breast feeding from affected mothers
- [ ] E has an increased incidence in Africa

7. HIV

- [ ] A may be diagnosed at birth by HIV antibody status
- [ ] B can present in infants with early onset AIDS
- [ ] C should be suspected if a low CD4 count is detected
- [ ] D may be diagnosed in infancy by p24 antigen
- [ ] E can be detected by polymerase chain reaction

8. Dysfunctions of the complement system include

- [ ] A recurrent viral infections with C1q deficiency
- [ ] B increased incidence of SLE with C1r deficiency
- [ ] C recurrent pneumococcal septicaemia with C2 deficiency
- [ ] D discoid lupus erythematosus with C2 deficiency
- [ ] E recurrent sinusitis with Factor D deficiency

9. Chronic granulomatous disease

- [ ] A does not occur in girls
- [ ] B is known to be X-linked
- [ ] C leads to increased viral infections
- [ ] D is suggested by a nitroblue tetrazolium test of 1
- [ ] E leads to increased staphylococcal infections

10. Chediak-Higashi syndrome

- [ ] A shows autosomal dominant inheritance
- [ ] B is usually associated with normal life expectancy
- [ ] C is associated with mental retardation
- [ ] D classically includes partial oculocutaneous albinism
- [ ] E has neutrophils with giant cytoplasmic granules

11. The following purpuric conditions are associated with normal platelet indices:

- [ ] A haemolytic uraemic syndrome
- [ ] B hereditary haemorrhagic telangiectasia
- [ ] C scurvy
- [ ] D Bernard-Soulier disease
- [ ] E Wiskott-Aldrich syndrome

12. A 5-year-old boy has Friedreich's ataxia:

- [ ] A his parents have a one in two chance of further affected children
- [ ] B he is likely to have ataxia as a later manifestation of this syndrome
- [ ] C his intelligence quotient will be lower than that of his normal siblings
- [ ] D he has an increased risk of developing diabetes mellitus
- [ ] E he will inevitably become blind as this is part of the syndrome

13. The causes of bilateral ophthalmoplegia include

- ☐ A brainstem glioma
- ☐ B chronic candidial meningitis
- ☐ C myasthenia gravis
- ☐ D atrial septal defect
- ☐ E posterior urethral valves

14. Hepatoblastomas

- ☐ A may present with calcification on abdominal X-ray
- ☐ B can present with sexual precocity
- ☐ C in over 60% of cases present with severe osteopenia
- ☐ D can present with an acute abdomen
- ☐ E in the majority of cases present in adolescence due to rupture of the mass

15. The Glasgow Coma scale

- ☐ A scores 2 for localizing a painful stimulus
- ☐ B scores 3 for eye opening to painful stimulus
- ☐ C scores 4 for an appropriate verbal response to questioning
- ☐ D scores 1 for decerebrate posturing
- ☐ E scores 1 for incomprehensible noises to verbal stimulus

16. The following is true of the catecholamine pathway and its components:

- ☐ A tyrosine is an amino acid with a 6 carbon ring structure
- ☐ B noradrenaline is formed from adrenaline by methylation of the terminal amine group
- ☐ C dopamine is converted to adrenaline by amidation of the central sulphur hydryl bond
- ☐ D the rate limiting step in the catecholamine synthetic pathway is the production of dihydroxyphenylalanine from tyrosine
- ☐ E tyrosine hydroxylase is inhibited by the presence of a large concentration of catecholamines

Practice Exam

17. The following drugs have been implicated in causing acute pancreatitis:

- ☐ A oestrogens
- ☐ B frusemide
- ☐ C sulphonamides
- ☐ D sodium valproate
- ☐ E tetracycline

18. The following side effects may be seen:

- ☐ A bronchoconstriction with non-steroidal anti-inflammatory drugs
- ☐ B papillary necrosis occurs with indomethacin
- ☐ C reversible abnormal liver function tests may arise with carbenicillin
- ☐ D renal tubular acidosis may be caused by amphotericin
- ☐ E peritoneal dialysis diminishes serum lithium levels

19. Ribavirin

- ☐ A is a nucleoside analogue
- ☐ B can only be given in aerosol formulation
- ☐ C is excreted predominantly in sweat
- ☐ D mainly acts to prevent viral entry into cells
- ☐ E resistance in vitro has been described

20. Cystic fibrosis

- ☐ A affects 1 in 10 000 children in the United Kingdom
- ☐ B may present with hepatic cirrhosis
- ☐ C has a median survival of 27-30 years
- ☐ D may be readily diagnosed by immunoreactive trypsin measurement to the age of 4 months
- ☐ E may present with pseudo-Bartter's syndrome

Practice Exam

21. Causes of nasal obstruction include

- [ ] A hypertrophic tonsils
- [ ] B dermoid cysts
- [ ] C Cruzon's syndrome
- [ ] D encephalocoele
- [ ] E tongue tie

22. The main differences between the adult and infant respiratory tracts are

- [ ] A the epiglottis of the infant is relatively inferior to the cervical vertebrae compared with that of the adult
- [ ] B the angle to the midline of the left main bronchus in the infant is the same as the angle of the right main bronchus
- [ ] C the infant has approximately 300 million alveoli
- [ ] D the surface area of the infant lung is half that of the adult
- [ ] E the tidal volume of the neonate is approximately 80 ml/kg body weight

23. Recognised complications of cystic fibrosis include

- [ ] A haemoptysis
- [ ] B intussusception
- [ ] C pilonidal sinus formation
- [ ] D portal hypertension
- [ ] E erythema marginatum

24. Regarding asthma

- [ ] A there is a decline in bronchial reactivity with the onset of puberty
- [ ] B puberty is more commonly delayed in atopic and asthmatic patients
- [ ] C short stature is expected in the majority of asthmatic patients
- [ ] D the majority of asthmatic children develop symptoms by the age of 5 years
- [ ] E recurrent wheeze may be caused by rhinovirus infection

25. The following may be associated with bronchiectasis

- ☐ A Kartagener's syndrome
- ☐ B allergic aspergillosis
- ☐ C Laurence-Moon-Biedl syndrome
- ☐ D aspiration of a foreign body
- ☐ E scimitar syndrome

26. Anorexia nervosa

- ☐ A has a 50% recovery rate with treatment
- ☐ B has a 5%-10% mortality rate
- ☐ C is increased in higher socio-economic classes
- ☐ D is associated with the male sex in 35% of cases
- ☐ E occurs exclusively in the age group 14–18 years

27. The INR is prolonged in

- ☐ A disseminated intravascular coagulation
- ☐ B hypofibrinogenaemia
- ☐ C factor XII deficency
- ☐ D vitamin C deficency
- ☐ E factor V deficency

28. The following are poor prognostic factors in ALL:

- ☐ A white count greater than 50 x 10^9/1
- ☐ B age less than 1 year
- ☐ C common ALL immunotype
- ☐ D 4:11 chromosomal translocation
- ☐ E 11:19 chromosomal translocation

29. Genetic causes of blindness include

- ☐ A retrolental fibroplasia
- ☐ B birth asphyxia
- ☐ C cortical blindness
- ☐ D Leber's amaurosis
- ☐ E Lawrence-Moon-Biedl syndrome

30. Causes of respiratory distress syndrome include

- ☐ A methaemoglobinaemia
- ☐ B meconium aspiration
- ☐ C transient tachypnoea of the newborn
- ☐ D pneumothorax
- ☐ E pulmonary haemorrhage

31. The following are associated with persistent fetal circulation syndrome:

- ☐ A birth asphyxia
- ☐ B maternal hyperthyroidism
- ☐ C congenital diaphragmatic hernia
- ☐ D respiratory alkalosis
- ☐ E pulmonary hypoplasia

32. The small for gestation baby has an increased incidence of the following problems when compared with an age-matched baby of appropriate weight:

- ☐ A polycythaemia
- ☐ B pulmonary haemorrhage
- ☐ C infection
- ☐ D increased incidence of congenital abnormalties
- ☐ E neutropenia

33. The following are strong indications for intubation:

- [ ] A stridor
- [ ] B Glasgow coma score of 11
- [ ] C absence of the gag reflex
- [ ] D central cyanosis
- [ ] E the development of unilateral pupillary dilation in a patient following head injury

34. Lymphomas are associated with the following X-linked disorders:

- [ ] A Bruton's agammaglobulinaemia
- [ ] B severe combined immunodeficiency syndrome (SCID)
- [ ] C coeliac disease
- [ ] D Di George's syndrome
- [ ] E Wiskott-Aldrich syndrome

35. Nephrotic syndrome

- [ ] A is characterised by reduced receptor mediated catabolism of cholesterol
- [ ] B is characterised by a decrease in procoagulant factors
- [ ] C is characterised by an increased susceptibility to infection
- [ ] D in children is most commonly due to focal glomerular sclerosis, which responds in the majority of cases to steroid treatment
- [ ] E may arise following infection with hepatitis B

36. The following hormones have the following influences:

- [ ] A gastrin alters gastric motility
- [ ] B enteroglucagon stimulates mucosal growth
- [ ] C motilin stimulates gastrointestinal motor activity
- [ ] D gastric inhibitory peptide inhibits insulin release
- [ ] E pancreatic polypeptide stimulates the release of gallbladder contents

Practice Exam

37. Causes of portal hypertension include

- ☐ A Budd-Chiari syndrome
- ☐ B eczema
- ☐ C schistosomiasis
- ☐ D alopecia
- ☐ E constrictive pericarditis

38. Gaucher's disease

- ☐ A results from accumulation of glucosylceramide
- ☐ B type II is associated with hepatosplenomegaly
- ☐ C is diagnosed by elevated levels of acid phosphatase
- ☐ D shows large lipid laden macrophage-like cells in the bone marrow
- ☐ E may be associated with multiple fractures in type 1 Gaucher's disease

39. Causes of systemic hypertension in the newborn include

- ☐ A raised intra-cranial pressure
- ☐ B coarctation of the aorta
- ☐ C renal vein thrombosis
- ☐ D congenital adrenal hyperplasia
- ☐ E infantile eczema

40. Maple syrup disease

- ☐ A in the severest form may present with ketoacidosis
- ☐ B has an increased anion gap
- ☐ C is associated with high CSF levels of leucine, isoleucine and valine
- ☐ D untreated may lead to cortical atrophy
- ☐ E requires a strict diet of cows' milk with an increased branched amino acid concentration

Practice Exam

41. In homocystinuria

- [ ] A aminoaciduria may abate with daily pyridoxine and folate
- [ ] B has upward lens dislocation as a common feature
- [ ] C hepatomegaly may be present
- [ ] D is associated with a normal intelligence quotient
- [ ] E is due to ornithine transcarbamylase deficiency

42. The following questions deal with cystinuria:

- [ ] A cystinuria is associated with elevated urinary lysine levels
- [ ] B with cystinuria there is an increased incidence of gallstones
- [ ] C elevated urinary cystine may be seen in Fanconi's syndrome
- [ ] D may have disturbed uptake of glycine in the bowel
- [ ] E acidification of the urine to below pH 5.1 will increase the solubility of cystine

43. Diet in chronic renal failure should

- [ ] A be high in carbohydrates
- [ ] B be low in fats
- [ ] C be high in protein
- [ ] D avoid excessive chocolate
- [ ] E allow only limited milk intake

44. In atrioseptal defects

- [ ] A the size of the shunt depends on the atrial pressure difference
- [ ] B the size of the shunt depends on the size of the defect
- [ ] C the size of the shunt depends on the compliance of the ventricles
- [ ] D pulmonary hypertension is common in childhood
- [ ] E atrial arrhythmias in adult life can occur

45. Coronary artery fistula

- ☐ A most often occurs in the left main descending branch
- ☐ B can cause angina
- ☐ C commonly gives rise to heart failure
- ☐ D may present with a continuous murmur
- ☐ E drains into the right heart in 10% of cases

46. Hashimoto thyroiditis may be associated with

- ☐ A Graves' disease
- ☐ B hyperparathyroidism
- ☐ C Schmidt syndrome
- ☐ D trisomy 21
- ☐ E Turner's syndrome

47. In Pendred syndrome

- ☐ A transmission is by autosomal dominant inheritance
- ☐ B hearing loss gradually develops
- ☐ C hearing loss is most pronounced at higher frequencies
- ☐ D goitre is usually large and present from birth
- ☐ E hypothyroidism is present from birth

48. A one-year-old girl presents to clinic with marked bilateral breast development

- ☐ A thelarche is very rare at this age
- ☐ B she is unlikely to have a benign condition
- ☐ C she will need active treatment
- ☐ D no investigations are required
- ☐ E this condition may be unilateral

49. Regarding diabetes

- [ ] A the somogyi effect is the term given to the erythematous colouring noted at a lipoatrophic injection site
- [ ] B HbA1c is an abnormal haemoglobin produced by the reduction of ferric ion
- [ ] C in ketoacidosis potassium restriction is required as circulating levels may be greatly elevated
- [ ] D in ketoacidosis 30-40 units/kg/hour of insulin are required
- [ ] E in ketoacidosis free fatty acid is metabolised in liver mitochondria to acetoacetyl CoA, acetoacetate and 3 hydroxybutyrate

50. Hypocalcaemia may be due to

- [ ] A pseudohypoparathyroidism
- [ ] B primary hypoparathyroidism
- [ ] C 1 hydroxylase deficiency in the vitamin D metabolic pathway
- [ ] D Fanconi's syndrome
- [ ] E Di George's syndrome

51. The following are causes of inappropiate ADH secretion:

- [ ] A tuberculosis
- [ ] B alopecia
- [ ] C hypothyroidism
- [ ] D eczema
- [ ] E Guillain-Barré syndrome

52. Pathological conditions which commonly lead to obesity include

- [ ] A Prader-Willi syndrome
- [ ] B hypothyroidism
- [ ] C Lawrence-Moon-Biedl syndrome
- [ ] D hypoparathyroidism
- [ ] E Klinefelter's syndrome

Practice Exam

53. The following are true of immunoglobulins:

- ☐ A IgA is involved in complement fixation
- ☐ B IgA forms immune complexes
- ☐ C IgM is involved in complement dependent lysis
- ☐ D IgM has a major role in agglutination
- ☐ E IgA plays a major part in complement dependent lysis

54. The following types of allergic reaction match the accompanying examples:

- ☐ A systemic lupus erythematosus and type III allergic reaction
- ☐ B graft versus host disease and type III allergic reaction
- ☐ C type II allergic reaction has an onset within days of a blood transfusion
- ☐ D acute anaphylactic response and type I allergic reaction
- ☐ E serum sickness and type IV allergic reaction

55. Systemic fungal infection in the neonate

- ☐ A may present with thrombocytopenia
- ☐ B is commoner in full term infants than in very low birthweight infants
- ☐ C can be diagnosed by fundoscopic inspection
- ☐ D joints are more commonly involved than the central nervous system
- ☐ E candidial hyphae from supra-pubic aspiration are of little consequence

56. Respiratory syncytial virus

- ☐ A is a DNA virus
- ☐ B is shed from the nose for up to 6 months following infection
- ☐ C causes outbreaks of infection in spring and summer time
- ☐ D antibody is present in 90% of children by 1 year of age
- ☐ E can lead to bronchiolitis obliterans

Practice Exam

57. The following are true:

☐ A capillary haemangiomata are always present from birth
☐ B capillary haemangiomata appear blue initially
☐ C cavernous haemangiomata may have a bruit
☐ D cavernous haemangiomata are associated with thrombocytopenia
☐ E haemangiomata can cause amblyopia

58. The following drugs may be used as specific antidotes to the accompanying intoxicating agents:

☐ A physiostigmine to reverse anticholinergic agents
☐ B nitric oxide for carbon monoxide poisoning
☐ C methanol for ethanol toxicity
☐ D N-acetyl cysteine for paracetamol overdose
☐ E desferrioxamine for iron overdosage

59. Common features of salicylate toxicity are

☐ A inappropiate ADH
☐ B cerebral oedema
☐ C non-cardiogenic pulmonary oedema
☐ D tinnitus
☐ E sweating

60. Pertussis immunisation

☐ A is contraindicated in subjects with neural tube defects
☐ B should not be given when there is a family history of allergy
☐ C should not be given when there is a family history of convulsions
☐ D should not be given if the previous immunisation produced a circumferential erythema at the site of the injection
☐ E gives rise to neurological complications more commonly than with the disease

PRACTICE EXAM ANSWERS

1. **D E**
   On cross-section of a normal kidney the medulla is within the cortex and the renal pyramids are located in the medulla layer. The renal pelvis is lined by transitional epithelium.
   The glomeruli, proximal tubules and distal tubules are found in the cortex, and the loops of Henlé and the collecting ducts extend down through the medulla.

2. **A B**
   Release of antidiuretic hormone in relation to plasma osmolality is controlled by the supraoptic and paraventricular areas of the hypothalamus. The lateral preoptic area responds to thirst.
   Antidiuretic hormone is primarily synthesised in the supraoptic region of the hypothalamus and transported bound to neurophysin along nerve axons to be stored in the neurohypophysis of the posterior pituitary.
   The biochemical structure in humans is 8-arginine vasopressin and in pigs 8-lysine vasopressin.
   Removal of antidiuretic hormone is via the liver and kidney, its plasma half-life being just 10–15 minutes.

3. **D E**
   Calcium is the most commonly found cation in the human body, but the majority is found in bones. Calcium homoeostasis is important for various reasons, especially for its effects on excitable tissue (nerve and muscle). The threshold potential varies inversely with plasma calcium concentration.
   In plasma two forms of calcium are found:
   1. Ionised calcium – about 1.25 mmol/l
   2. Bound calcium – about 1.25 mmol/l.
   Only the ionised calcium is filtered by the kidney. Reabsorption occurs throughout each portion of the nephron. In the loop of Henlé calcium is absorbed from the ascending limb, this process is inhibited by frusemide. Only about 5% of the filtered load is lost in the urine. This is usually counter balanced by daily intake.

4. **ALL FALSE**
   C3 levels are reduced in acute poststreptococcal glomerulonephritis and membranoproliferative glomerulonephritis, they are normal in membranous glomerulonephritis, rapidly progressive (crescentic) glomerulonephritis, Goodpasture's disease and Henoch-Schonlein purpura.

5. **A C D E**
   Infantile polycystic disease is an autosomally recessive inherited condition classically with cysts in the kidney and liver. There are numerous cysts located in the cortex and medulla of the kidney, which cause

Practice Exam Answers

dilatations of the collecting ducts. These lead to interstitial fibrosis, tubular atrophy and progressive renal failure.

The liver involvement also varies in severity. Cirrhosis, portal hypertension and bleeding oesophageal varices may occur.

Presentation is commonly at birth with bilateral flank masses. Severe cases with oligohydramnios lead to kidney and lung damage and classical features of Potter's syndrome. Later presentation may be with nephrogenic diabetes insipidus, renal failure or hypertension.

Diagnosis is important not only for early treatment but also for the genetic counselling required.

6. **B D E**

Vertical transmission of HIV infection from mother to infant may occur at any time before, during or after delivery. There are higher rates of transmission in Africa than in the United Kingdom possibly due to different types of HIV subgroups. Factors associated with increased risk include maternal p24 HIV antigen, a low maternal CD4 count, breast feeding and delivery before 34 weeks. Current recommendations are that although breast feeding has been shown to increase risk of HIV the morbidity and mortality in developing countries of not breast feeding make stopping a more dangerous option. Accordingly the World Health Organisation recommends continued breast feeding in developing countries.

7. **B C D E**

HIV infection in neonates has previously been difficult to detect as maternal antibodies remain until 18 months of age. Diagnosis is possible if AIDS occurs early on, p24 antigen is detected in peripheral blood or a positive polymerase chain reaction is seen. Reduced CD4 count and raised immunoglobulins should raise suspicion.

8. **B C D E**

Dysfunctions of the complement system are associated with collagen-vascular disease and recurrent bacterial infections, often meningococcal and pneumococcal. Deficiencies to varying degrees are often found in families. Compensation occasionally occurs if the deficiencies can be counteracted by the alternative pathway.

9. **B E**

Chronic granulomatous disease is a condition of defective neutrophil function leading to an increase in bacterial and fungal infections. It is felt to be X-linked but 20% of cases occur in girls, either due to an autosomal recessive form or possibly excessive lyonisation. Classically defective neutrophil function can be detected by the nitroblue tetrazolium test which will be 0 in chronic granulomatous disease. Bacteria

Practice Exam Answers

are normally phagocytosed but cannot be lysed, therefore ingested microbes cannot be killed, leading to persistence of infection.

10. **C D E**
    Chediak-Higashi syndrome follows autosomal recessive inheritance. It is characterised by:
    - recurrent infections
    - neutrophils with giant cytoplasmic granules, with defective chemotaxis, degranulation and intracellular killing
    - partial oculocutaneous albinism, photophobia and nystagmus.

    Symptoms usually develop in early childhood with death by 10 years from infection or malignancy. Neurological abnormalities can develop including mental retardation, long tract signs, cerebellar involvement and peripheral neuropathies.

11. **B C**
    Other conditions of purpura with normal platelet indices include Henoch-Schonlein purpura, infections with coxsackie, rubella and Ehlers-Danlos.

    Haemolytic uraemic syndrome is characterised by microangiopathy giving rise to low platelet counts.

    Wiskott-Aldrich syndrome comprises small platelets with normal megakaryocytes, eczema and defective lymphocyte function. This condition is inherited in an X-linked manner.

    Bernard-Soulier syndrome is caused by a deficency of membrane glycoprotein 1. This autosomal recessive disorder is characterised by chronic purpura and bruising, and low platelet counts of large volume.

12. **D**
    Friedreich's ataxia is an autosomal recessive condition, with an onset between 3 to 17 years. This condition commonly presents with ataxia as a prominent feature. Later in the disease dysarthria, pyramidal signs and posterior column loss are noted. The intelligence quotient is unaffected.

    There is an increased incidence of diabetes mellitus and cardiomyopathy. One quarter of the patients develop optic atrophy but of these only two-thirds will develop reduced visual acuity.

13. **A B C**
    Other causes include congenital myopathies, myotonia dystrophica and thyrotoxicosis.

    Bilateral ptosis may be familial, inherited in an autosomal dominant fashion. It is also associated with Turner's syndrome and trisomies 13 and 18. Bilateral ptosis may also be seen with Moebius syndrome, Alpert's syndrome and Smith-Lemli-Opitz syndrome.

14. A B D

Hepatoblastomas may present with sexual precocity often with highly elevated beta HCG. In about 30% of cases is there severe osteopenia which may be associated with vertrebral fractures.

Rupture of the mass occurs in infancy.

15. ALL FALSE

The **Glasgow coma scale** has been validated for use up to the age of 4 years.

It scores the best response obtained in terms of verbal response, eye opening and motor response.

Eye Opening	Score
No response	1
Response to pain	2
Response to voice	3
Spontaneous	4

Verbal Response	Score
No response	1
Incomprehensible sounds	2
Inappropiate words	3
Disorientated conversation	4
Orientated and appropiate talk	5

Motor Response	Score
No response	1
Decerebrate posturing	2
Decorticate posturing	3
Flexion withdrawal	4
Localizes pain	5
Obeys commands	6

A score of less than 9 suggests severe injury and a score of 8 or less would indicate the need for intubation and ventilation.

16. A D E

Tyrosine is an amino acid which is hydroxylated to form 3,4 dihydroxyphenylalanine. This in turn is decarboxylated to give dopamine. Dopamine beta hydroxylase inserts a hydroxyl group into the methyl group of dopamine to produce noradrenaline. Methylation of the terminal amine group changes noradrenaline into adrenaline.

Catecholamine in large quantities inhibits tyrosine hydroxylase, hence the rate of production is controlled by a process of negative feedback.

Practice Exam Answers

17. **A B C D E**
Other drugs which cause acute pancreatitis include L-asparaginase, azathioprine, chlorothiazides, steroids, and intravenous parenteral nutrition.

18. **A B C D E**
Bronchoconstriction is seen with aspirin as well as with other non-steroidal anti-inflammatory agents. These agents can also induce rhinitis.
The underlying mechanism probably relates to the relative rates of synthesis (by enzymatic processes) of prostaglandins with inhibition of cyclo-oxygenase and increasing the 5 lipo-oxygenase pathway producing an excess of bronchoconstricting leukotrienes, LTC4, LTD4 and LTE4. There may be a dose dependent effect, that is at lower doses no such bronchoconstricting or rhinitic effect is seen.
Non-steroidal anti-inflammatory effects also include renal impairment, by depletion of prostaglandins within the kidney. These prostaglandins ordinarily provide protection against the effects of anti-diuretic hormone and the renin-angiotensin system, both of which have a renal vasoconstrictive effect.

19. **A**
Ribavirin is a nucleoside analogue, with three postulated modes of action, these being to decrease intracellular GTP guanosine leading to suppressed production, causing abnormal RNA to be formed, and it may cause a direct suppressive effect on viral polymerase, thus inhibiting replication.
Ribavirin may be given orally, or by intravenous injection and is effective in a number of RNA and DNA viral illnesses. It is largely excreted in the urine, with a lesser quantity being lost in the stool.

20. **B C E**
Cystic fibrosis has a heterozygous carriage rate of 1 in 20 caucasians in the United Kingdom with an incidence of 1 in 2500.
It may present with neonatal intestinal obstruction giving rise to meconium ileus. Older children may develop the meconium ileus equivalent syndrome. Pancreatic duct obstruction may lead to pancreatic deficiency and failure to thrive. Obstruction of the biliary tree may lead to hepatic cirrhosis. Male fertility may be affected as the development of the Wolffian duct system may be abnormal.
Electrolyte imbalance may also occur with excessive loss of sodium chloride in sweat with secondary hypokalaemia developing as an attempt to conserve sodium loss. This setting is better known as pseudo-Bartter's syndrome.
With improved management of patients with cystic fibrosis the median age of survival has risen and may continue to improve.
The gold standard remains the sweat test; immunoreactive trypsin is elevated in the first 2 weeks of life following pancreatic damage which has occurred in utero. This test however loses its specificity

Practice Exam Answers

after 6 weeks of life. This test is unreliable in neonates surgically treated for meconium ileus.

21. **B C D**
Adenotonsillar hypertrophy may cause upper airway obstruction.
Other causes include choanal atresia, choanal stenosis, midline hypoplasia as seen in craniosynostoses such as Apert's syndrome or Cruzon's syndrome or masses such as dermoid cysts, tumours and encephalocoeles.

22. **ALL FALSE**
The epiglottis of the infant is relatively superior and anteriorly placed compared with that of the adult.
The right main bronchus has a steeper angle, towards the midline, compared with the left main bronchus, hence the tendency for foreign bodies to lodge in the right main bronchus.
At birth the neonate has roughly 24 million alveoli. At the age of 8, there has been a 10-fold increase to 240 million. The adult lung is estimated to contain 280 million.
The surface area of the newborn's lung is approximately 2.8 m^2, increasing to 35 m^2 by the age of 8, with the normal adult lung being some 75 m^2.
The tidal volume of the neonate is of the order of 6-8 ml/kg body weight.

23. **A B D**
Recognised complications of cystic fibrosis include:

Respiratory
Infections
Pneumothorax
Haemoptysis
Nasal polyposis
Allergic aspergillosis

Cardiovascular
Pulmonary hypertension
Cor pulmonale

Gastrointestinal
Rectal prolapse
Cirrhosis
Portal hypertension
Hypersplenism
Cholecystitis
Gall stones
Biliary stricture

Practice Exam Answers

Pancreatitis
Intussusception

Other
Diabetes mellitus
Male infertility
Hypertrophic pulmonary osteoarthropathy
Arthropathy

Modes of presentation of cystic fibrosis

Well recognised modes in neonates
Meconium ileus
Prolonged jaundice
Positive screening (eg immunoreactive trypsin)

Other modes of presentation
Recurrent cough or wheeze
Offensive loose stools
Slow weight gain / failure to thrive
Salty when kissed
Nasal polyposis
Rectal prolapse
Heat prostration in hot weather- pseudo-Bartter's syndrome

24. A B D E
Only severely affected asthmatics fail to reach expected height. Wheeziness may also follow infection with respiratory synctial virus as in bronchiolitis. Children who do not have an atopic element tend to outgrow their wheeziness by primary school age.

25. A B D E
Kartagener's syndrome comprises ciliary dyskinesia with sinusitis, male/female infertility, dextrocardia.

Allergic aspergillosis may cause bronchiectasis as may the prolonged presence of an inhaled foreign body. Cystic fibrosis may also be associated with bronchiectasis.

Scimitar syndrome is the association of a hypoplastic right lung with the systemic arterial supply and anomalous venous drainage.

26. A B C
This is most often seen in adolescent girls, with only 5–10% of cases occurring in males; however anorexia nervosa can present at any age. Family dynamics play an important part in the aetiology, with a rigid tight knit family and an overintrusive relationship with the female parent.

There is an increasing incidence in higher socio-economic class.

25% of cases improve to the extent that the eating disorder subdues, and the remainder continue to run a persistent course.

Practice Exam Answers

27. **A B E**
Prothrombin time may be prolonged due to deficiencies in factors V, VII and X, to prothrombin deficiency, hypofibrinogenaemia, liver disease, vitamin K deficiency or in acquired coagulation states such as nephrotic syndrome or disseminated intravascular coagulation.

28. **A B D E**
Other poor prognostic features include B cell type and CNS disease at diagnosis. Good prognostic factors are white cell count under 20 x 10⁹/1, age between 2 to 5 years, and common ALL immunotype.

29. **D E**
Other inheritable causes of blindness are congenital cataracts, anophthalmos and retinitis pigmentosa.

30. **B C D E**
Other causes include upper airway obstruction, hyaline membrane disease, pneumonia, pulmonary hypoplasia, pulmonary cystic disease, persistent fetal circulation, heart failure, congenital diaphragmatic hernia, and neuromuscular disorders such as myopathies.

31. **A C E**
Metabolic acidosis, antenatal hypoxia with fetal distress, hyaline membrane disease, congenital pneumonia, hypothermia, hypoglycaemia and infection such as group B streptococcal infection are clinically associated conditions.

32. **A D E**
There is no increased incidence of pulmonary haemorrhage or infection. There is an increased incidence of 3–6% of congenital abnormalities such as Potter's syndrome and chromosomal abnormalities. Neutropenia and thrombocytopenia are more common especially if the weight is below 1 kilogram. In the small for gestational age baby the liver glycogen stores are less hence there is a increased incidence of hypoglycaemia.

33. **C E**
The major indicators for intubation are:
1. The inability to maintain a patent airway despite airway opening techniques
2. A Glasgow coma score of 8 or lower: if the patient exhibits a rapidly deteriorating score, for example 11 dropping to 9 within a short period of time, intubation may be considered
3. An absence of cough or gag reflexes portend the inability to protect the airway
4. Hypoventilation/hypoxia
5. Impending herniation of the brain.

Practice Exam Answers

34. **A B E**

    Coeliac disease is associated with intestinal lymphomas but is not inherited in an X-linked manner. Di George's syndrome is linked with oral malignancies and with CNS tumours but not with lymphomas. IgA deficency is linked with lymphomas but is probably inherited in an autosomal dominant fashion.

35. **C E**

    There is an overall reduction in the catabolism of cholesterol as well as an associated decrease in its synthesis.

    Procoagulant factors are increased and there is a decrease in the thrombolytic capacity hence the increased incidence of arterial and venous thromboses in nephrotic syndrome.

    By far the commonest cause of nephrotic syndrome in children is minimal change glomerulonephritis, which on the whole responds to steroid treatment.

    Hepatitis B and secondary syphilis are recognised to give rise to nephrotic syndrome. Other causative agents include drugs such as gold, penicillamine, captopril, systemic lupus erthymatosus and tumours.

    Secondary causes of distal RTA are nephrocalcinosis, vitamin D intoxication, Ehlers-Danlos syndrome, primary hyperparathyroidism.

36. **A B C E**

Gastrin	increases gastric acid secretion
	increases gastric motility
Cholccystokinin	increases bicarbonate from the pancreas
Motilin	increases gastrointestinal activity
Gastric inhibitory peptide	increases insulin release
Enteroglucagon	increases mucosal growth
Pancreatic polypeptide	inhibits pancreatic enzyme and stimulates gallbladder contraction

37. **A C E**

    Prehepatic causes:
    Following umbilical venous cannulization
    Phlebitis of the portal vein
    Extrinsic compression eg due to pancreas, tumour, lymphadenopathy in the porta hepatis
    Hepatic causes
    Cirrhosis
    Schistosomiasis
    Gaucher's disease
    Hodgkin's disease
    Portal fibrosis
    Felty's syndrome

Posthepatic causes
    Budd-Chiari syndrome
    Inferior vena cava obstruction
Cardiac causes
    constrictive pericarditis
    right atrial myxoma

38. A B D E

There are three forms of Gaucher's disease, all due to a deficiency of glucosylceramide beta-glucosidase activity leading to the accumulation of glucosylceramide.

Type 1 is a chronic non-neuropathic form and may present in late childhood or adulthood with hepatosplenomegaly and features of hypersplenism. Bone infiltration can occur giving rise to osteopenia and fractures.

Type 2 is an acute neuropathic form, presenting in the first few months of life. Hepatosplenomegaly and brain stem involvement are seen with increasing spasticity, brisk reflexes and failure to thrive due to feeding difficulties. Death usually occurs in the first year of life.

Type 3 is a subacute neuropathic form with onset around 1 year. Neurological involvement is not as extensive as type 2 but all cases have splenomegaly. Hepatomegaly is also commmonly seen.

The diagnosis is made by assaying the activity of beta-glucosidase in leucocytes or in skin fibroblasts.

Acid phosphatase is very often elevated but this is not diagnostic.

39. A B C D

Causes of hypertension in the neonate:
Cardiovascular
    Coarctation of the aorta
    Renal
    Renal vein thrombosis
    Renal parenchymal infection
    Renal failure
    Dysplastic/polycystic renal disorder
    Urinary tract obstruction
Endocrine
    Congenital adrenal hyperplasia
    Hyperthyroidism
    Hyperaldosteronism
CNS
    Raised intracranial pressure
Drugs
    Steroid therapy
    Methylxanthines

Practice Exam Answers

40. A B C D
Maple syrup urine disease affects the metabolism of branched chain amino acids, namely valine, isoleucine and leucine, giving rise to elevated urinary and plasma levels. Increased levels are also found in the CSF. Patients may be only intermittently affected; some forms respond to thiamine treatment. In the severest form, convulsions, hypoglycaemia, an increased anion gap and ketoacidosis occur, leading rapidly to death. The diagnosis can be made by assaying white blood cells or fibroblast enzyme activity. Dietary treatment is an absolute requirement. Survivors if untreated may become severely disabled.

41. A C
Classically this condition is due to cystathionine synthetase deficiency producing a clinical picture similar to Marfan's syndrome, with arachnodactyly and long limbs. There is however no joint hypermobility. Features common only to homocystinuria include downward dislocation of the lens (upward in Marfan's), an increased incidence of intravascular thromboses and osteoporosis.

Hepatomegaly is due to fatty enlargement and over 50% have significant development delay.

About 1 in 200 people are heterozygote carriers for this autosomal recessive disorder. If there is no response to vitamin supplementation, a low methionine diet is usually commenced.

42. A C
Cystinuria is characterised by increased urinary levels of cystine, ornithine, arginine and lysine. The uptake of these amino acids is also reduced in the bowel.

There is an increased incidence of renal calculi (not gallstones) and alkalinisation of the urine increases the solubility of excreted cystine. Penicillamine has also been used to increase its solubility and reduce the incidence of stone formation.

43. A D E
The diet in chronic renal failure should contain maximum calorie intake, mainly via carbohydrates and fats, especially medium chain triglycerides. Proteins are of less value and recommended in a form easily metabolised to usable amino acids. Build up of nitrogenous waste can lead to symptoms of nausea and anorexia.

Substances high in potassium should be avoided, for example, bananas, chocolate, crisps, spinach and other greens. Further high phosphate containing foods should be avoided, such as milk, yoghurt and cheese. It is often difficult to avoid such basic foods as dairy products so a phosphate binding agent is frequently added to the therapy.

Practice Exam Answers

Secondary to inadequate intake children may become deficient in water soluble vitamins which need replacing. Fat soluble vitamins do not become deficient.

44. B C E
The size of the shunt in atrioseptal defects is dependent on the size of the defect and the compliance of the ventricles. In infancy the pulmonary vascular resistance is initially high and gradually reduces, hence significant shunting may take months or even years to develop. Pulmonary hypertension is generally only seen in adult life. Other changes such as right atrial and ventricular hypertrophy also tend to be seen in adulthood: the enlargement of the atria giving rise to arrhythmias. Abnormal sinus node and atrioventricular node dysfunction can be seen in children.

45. B D
Coronary artery fistulae involve the right coronary artery most commonly, with 90% of the fistulae draining into the right heart. Large fistulae may cause reduced exercise capacity, shortness of breath or angina. A continuous murmur may be audible. Heart failure is an uncommon feature. Diagnosis may be made by echocardiography if the fistula is particularly large; otherwise definitive diagnosis is reached by aortography or selective coronary artery arteriography. Surgical ligation is recommended as complications such as myocardial infarction, arrhythmia, thrombosis and rupture can occur.

46. A C D E
Hashimoto thyroiditis or lymphocytic thyroiditis is the most common cause of thyroid disease in children and adolescents. It is the most common cause of juvenile hypothyroidism (with or without goitre). The incidence may be as high as 1% in schoolchildren.

Hashimoto thyroiditis is an organ specific autoimmune disease. The condition is up to seven times more common in girls than boys. Onset is generally after six years of age and peaks in adolescence. Goitres tend to be non-tender and diffuse.

There is often transient hyperthyroidism in symptomatic patients followed by hypothyroidism. Spontaneous remission may occur.

Schmidt syndrome or Type 2 polyglandular autoimmune disease comprises Addison's disease with insulin dependent diabetes mellitus and autoimmune thyroid disease such as Hashimoto thyroiditis.

Autoimmune thyroid disease may also be associated with hypoparathyroidism, pernicious anaemia, vitiligo and/or alopecia and it has an increased incidence in children with congenital rubella. It may be associated with chromosomal abnormalities eg. Turner's syndrome and Down's syndrome.

Practice Exam Answers

47. C

Pendred syndrome is a congenital condition comprising deafness and goitre. It is transmitted by autosomal recessive inheritance. Hearing loss tends to be severe and present from birth, being most pronounced in the higher frequencies.

The goitre generally appears at puberty or later, although it may be present in early childhood. The goitre is soft and diffuse, gradually becoming nodular in adult life. Patients are initially euthyroid but may progress to become hypothyroid.

Lifelong treatment with thyroid hormone is required in hypothyroid patients.

48. E

Benign premature thelarche is the isolated appearance of unilateral or bilateral breast tissue in girls aged six months to two years. No other signs of puberty should be present and there should be no evidence of the effects of oestrogens eg. thickening of the vaginal mucosa or bone age acceleration.

Ingestion or application of oestrogen containing compounds must be excluded.

It is advisable to carry out pelvic ultrasound to ensure no ovarian pathology. Also FSH, LH and oestradiol plasma levels should be measured to exclude hypothalmic-pituitary-ovarian dysfunction.

Follow up is usually for six to twelve months to ensure no signs of precocious puberty develop.

The prognosis is excellent as the majority of cases regress and no treatment is usually necessary.

49. E

The Somogyi effect is the term given to the effects seen when an excess of intermediate acting insulin is given in the evening dose. This causes an overnight hypoglycaemia and ketone formation with subsequent rebound hyperglycaemia, hence a morning urine sample on testing shows the presence of ketone bodies as well as glucose. The necessary treatment is not to increase the quantity of insulin but to alter the balance of long term and intermediate insulin prescribed for the evening dose.

HbA1c arises as a consequence of glycsolation of the N-terminal valine indicating serum glucose levels over the past 2-3 months.

In diabetic ketoacidosis there is total depletion of intracellular potassium, hence there is an overall depletion of body potassium despite an apparently normal serum potassium level.

In the treatment of diabetic ketoacidosis, small quantities of insulin are required, typically of the order of 0.1–0.25 units/kg/hour. Careful attention to the correction of hypovolaemia and electrolyte disturbance is mandatory in order to ensure a full recovery. Hyperglycaemia gives rise to a massive osmotic diuresis causing a peripheral vasoconstriction, tissue hypoperfusion and the subsequent development of anaerobic metabolic and the generation of lactic acidosis.

50. **A B C D E**
Hypocalcaemia is seen in:

1. Dietary imbalances:
   a). vitamin D deficiency
   b). calcium deficiency
   c). excessive phytate ingestion
2. Renal disorders such as:
   a). renal tubular acidosis
   b). tubular disorders eg. Fanconi's
   c). hypophosphataemic rickets
   d). familial vitamin D resistant rickets
   e). vitamin D resistant rickets
3. Vitamin D deficiency states as seen in:
   a). malabsorption
   b). liver disease
   c). uraemia
   d). anticonvulsant therapy
   e). enzyme disorders in vitamin D metabolism
4. Alkalosis
   a). an excess of alkali agents
   b). pyloric stenosis
   c). hyperventilation
5. Hypoparathyroidism is associated with low calcium and low parathyroid hormone levels. This occurs sporadically, or can be familial. Hypoparathyroidism due to aplasia is associated with Di George syndrome.
6. Pseudohypoparathyroidism is associated with low calcium but normal parathyroid hormone levels.

51. **A C E**
   Causes of inappropriate ADH secretion
   CNS: meningitis/encephalitis
         trauma
         hypoxia
         haemorrhage
         congenital malformation
         Gullian-Barré

Practice Exam Answers

Respiratory: pneumonia
tuberculosis
asthma
pneumothorax
cystic fibrosis

Endocrine: hypothyroidism
adrenocortical dysfunction
hypoglycaemia

Postoperatively
Drugs such as analgesics

Malignancy
Trauma and burns

52. B C E A
Other causes of obesity are:
chromosomal – trisomy 21
pseudohypoparathyroidism
hypothyroidism
growth hormone deficency
Cushing's syndrome
cerebral disorders such as hydrocephalus, craniopharyngioma, trauma, infection such as menigo/encephalitis.

53. C D

Reaction	IgG	IgA	IgM
Precipitation	+	+	++
Agglutination	+	+	+
Complement fixation	+++	-	+
Complement dependent fixation	+	-	+++
Immune complex fixation	+	-	+

54. A D

Type I reaction is mediated by the liberation from tissue mast cells of histamine, bradykinin and other inflammatory mediators, producing an effect within a few minutes. Examples of this reaction include acute anaphylaxis, hay fever, asthma, urticaria and food and drug allergies.

Type II is a cytotoxic reaction, enforced by circulating antibody such as IgG or IgM which reacts to cell surface bound antigen causing lysis in the presence of complement. Drug induced reactions are an example as are rhesus, ABO isoimmunisation and blood transfusion reactions. These reactions in sensitised individuals may take from minutes to hours to manifest.

Type III is due to circulating immune complexes of combined antigen and antibody forming microprecipitates and lodging in the microvasculature. Onset of this reaction may take a few hours to days, with Henoch-Schonlein purpura, serum sickness, poststreptococcal nephritis and systemic lupus erythematosus being recognised examples.

Type IV is due to cell mediated (or delayed hypersensitivity) reaction, wherein sensitised lymphocytes reacting with antigen evoke a cytokine response to induce lymphocyte migration. This is seen in eczema, graft versus host disease and with tuberculin testing.

55. A C

Very low birthweight babies and even babies which are smaller than average are at high risk of systemic fungal infection. At an increased risk are babies who have been on long term broad spread antibiotics, have required intravenous access for total parenteral nutrition or who are immunocompromised.

Presentation may be with respiratory depression, apnoea, bradycardia, temperature instability, low or elevated white cell count, raised platelet count, glucose intolerance or a combination of these features.

The central nervous system and uro-genital tracts are particularly affected by fungal septicaemia, hence the presence of hyphae in urine obtained by suprapubic aspiration is highly significant. Joint involvement is not as commonly seen.

Fundoscopy is useful to reveal endophthalmitis.

56. E

RSV is a RNA virus, has an incubation period of 3 days and is shed for up to 27 days from the nasal mucosa following infection. It is the major cause of bronchiolitis in children with outbreaks occurring from late autumn to early spring.

By the age of 3 almost all children have neutralising antibodies which last for 6–9 months.

At particular risk are infants with congenital heart disease, bronchopulmonary dysplasia or who are immunocompromised.

These groups have mortality rates of up to 37 per 100, whereas the mortality rate in normal infants is less than 1%. Other complications include pneumothorax, atelectasis and the development of bronchiolitis obliterans.

57. C D E

Capillary naevi tend to appear in the first few weeks of life as an area of paleness followed by telangiectasia. Growth of the superficial capillaries continues rapidly for the first few months of life and then slows and stops by 10 months of age. Involution occurs after an indefinite static phase, with the mass becoming softer and grey. The majority of cases will have disappeared by the age of 5.

Cavernous haemangiomata may extend to involve the epidermis or may not be visible. With large arteriovenous malformations within the haemangioma a bruit may be heard. Platelet consumption may also be a feature, this being called the Kasabach Merritt syndrome.

Haemangiomata can cause amblyopia if they close the eyelid, preventing visual development.

58. A D E

Carbon monoxide is treated by oxygen including hyperbaric oxygen treatment.

Methanol overdose can be combatted by giving ethanol.

Supportive treatment is integral to treating all these overdoses.

Dialysis may be useful in ethanol and methanol toxicity.

59. D E

Common features	Uncommon features
pyrexia	haemolysis
sweating	renal failure
nausea	liver failure
vomiting	respiratory depression
coagulopathy	inappropriate ADH secretion
fits	cerebral
coma	non-cardiogenic pulmonary oedema
tinnitus	
increased respiratory rate	

60. D

Contraindications are local and general:

Local If with the previous injection there has been an extensive area of redness and swelling involving the antero-lateral aspect of the thigh if given in the leg or the majority of the circumference of the arm.

General Anaphylaxis, bronchospasm, laryngeal oedema, fever of 39.5 degrees Centigrade within 48 hours of vaccination, collapse, convulsions or encephalopathy within 72 hours.

The incidence of neurological disorders is higher following the illness than following immunisation.

Stable neurological disorders, a family history of convulsions or allergy are not contraindications.

APPENDIX: REVISION LISTS

Abilities at 6 months of age 128
ADH secretion, causes of inappropriate 220
Adrenal glucocorticoids, peripheral actions 12
AIDS, indications of 151
Amino acids, essential 15
Apgar scores 51
Autoimmune polyglandular syndromes 110
Blood in stools in neonatal period, causes 96
Blood pressure and saturation in the heart 79
Bone marrow transplantation 65
Breast milk, constituents 39
Bronchiectasis, associated conditions 60
Cataracts, associated conditions 132
cDNA probes, conditions suitable for 110
Chromosomal locations associated with diseases 163
Coagulation pathways 68
Colobomata of the iris, associated conditions 132
Common carotid artery, relations 4
Congenital toxoplasmosis 149
Congenital rubella syndrome, features of 148
Cyanosis and pulmonary markings 81
Cystic fibrosis, complications 212
Death in childhood, causes 169
Disordered fetal swallowing 52
DNA-containing viruses 150
Drugs which increase LOP 27
Drugs which decrease LOP 28
Eisenmenger's syndrome 79
Electrolyte concentrations in body compartments 95
Emergency management of supraventricular tachycardia and shock 81
Energy requirement (kcal/day) by age 39
Erythema nodosum, infective causes 158
Fibrosis, upper/lower lobe 58
Glasgow coma scale 210
Glucagon, actions 12
Glycolysis, stages 21
Heaf test 174
Hearing investigations, indications for 128
Hodgkin's disease, histological types 73
Hypercalcaemia, causes 109
Hypertension in the neonate, causes 213
Hypocalcaemia 219
Hypokalaemic metabolic acidosis, causes 89

Hypomanic/manic episodes, causes of 187
IgG, IgA, IgM 221
Increased permeability, causes 97
Incubation times of infectious diseases 147
Insulin, effects 21
Internal jugular vein, posterior relations 5
Intubation, indications for 214
Iron count, causes of low 65
Kawasaki, diagnostic criteria 150
Liver, main roles 17
Macrocephaly and microcephaly 125
Mucopolysaccharidoses 103
Notifiable diseases 147
Obesity, causes of 220
Oesophagus, relations 3
Organ donation, contraindications 190
Pancreatitis, causes 96
Pauciarticular arthritis 139
Pertussis immunisation, contraindications 223
Polyarthritic rheumatoid arthritis 138
Polyhydramnios, associated conditions 52
Polyp/glioma/encephalocoele/dermoid 44
Portal hypertension, causes 215
Protein requirement (g/day) by age 39
Pseudohermaphroditism, syndromes linked with 110
Raised neutrophil count, non-infective causes 66
Renal tubular acidosis, secondary causes 87
Rheumatic fever, criteria for diagnosis 80
Rickets and hypoparathyroidism 112
Salicylate toxicity, features of 223
Septic arthritis, organisms causing 151
Skeletal abnormalities of Down's syndrome and Down's syndrome 163
SLE, categories 85
Stridor, causes 61
Stridor, persistent/acute causes 58
Teratogens 52
Thyroid binding globulins, causes of altered levels 113
Transudative ascitic fluid collection, causes 96
Urinary tract infections, management 88
Vitamins 39
VZIG, recommended uses 175
Wheezing, causes 61
Wilms' tumour, stages 74
X-linked recessive disorders 162

INDEX

Page numbers given are for pages on which relevant questions appear. The word shown may not always be used in the question but may appear in the explanatory answer.

Abetalipoproteinaemia 90, 29
Achondroplasia 106, 119, 130, 136
Active metabolites 24
Acute epiglottis 57
Acute hepatitis 108
Acute lymphoblastic leukaemia 69
Acute otitis media 41
Addison's disease 84, 105
Adenomatoid lung malformation, congenital 55
Adenotonsillectomy 41
Adenovirus 145
ADH 204, 206
Adrenal glucocorticoids 6
Adrenal hyperplasia, congenital 106, 108, 144, 201
Adrenaline 188
AIDS 146
Alagille's syndrome 117
Aldosterone 7
ALL 69, 198
Alpert's syndrome 195
Alpha-1-antitrypsin deficiency 55, 92
Alpha-fetoprotein 84, 115
Alpha-fetoprotein, serum 45
Alport syndrome 82
Amino acid disorders 38
Amino acids, essential 10, 19
Aminoglycosides 24, 46
Anaemia 62
Anaemia, aplastic 62
Anaemia, leucoerythroblastic 69
Anaphylaxis 57, 172, 205, 206
Angio-oedema, hereditary 34
Anorexia nervosa 182, 183, 198
Anthrax 143
Antidiuretic hormone 192
Antituberculous drugs 183
Aortic stenosis 76
Aortopulmonary window 75
Apgar score 47
Aplastic anaemia 62
Apnoea 45, 47, 54, 105
Appendicitis 93
Apt test 91
Artery, common carotid 1
Ascitic fluids 92

Asphyxiating thoracic dystrophy 136
Asthma 54, 154, 197, 204
Ataxia 99, 115, 116, 118, 181
Ataxia telangiectasia 115, 159
Atopic eczema 154
Atrial septal defect 76, 77, 195
Atrioseptal defect 75, 202
Atrioventricular canal defects 75
Attributable risk 167
Atypical mononuclear cells 63
Autism 183
Autosomal disorders 159

B cell defects 33, 161
B12 38, 90
B2 37
B6 37, 99
Bacillus cereus 144
Bartter's syndrome 84
Battery, swallowed 23
BCG 45, 171, 172
Beckwith-Wiedemann syndrome 177
Benign murmurs 75
Berger's nephropathy 82
Bernard-Soulier syndrome 63, 194
Beta thalassaemia 62
Bile salts 10
Biotin deficiency 99
Bipolar illness 181
Birth asphyxia 199
Blind loop syndrome 90
Blindness 118, 130, 199
Bloom's syndrome 154
"Blueberry muffin" 69
Bone marrow transplantation 62
Borrelia burgdorferi 146
Brachial plexus injuries 46
Breast feeding 24
Bronchiectasis 56
Bronchiolitis 54, 57, 62, 205
Bruton's agammaglobulinaemia 200
Budd-Chiari syndrome 201

Calcium 101, 192
Candidiasis, chronic mucocutaneous 62, 106
Carbamazepine 181, 182
Carcinoid 93

225

Index

Cardiac catheterisation 75
Cardiomyopathy, hypertrophic 48
Cardiomyopathy 70, 194
Cataracts 29, 100, 105, 106, 114, 130, 160, 198
Catecholamine pathway 195
cDNA 106
Cells, atypical mononuclear 63
CHARGE syndrome 130
Chediak-Higashi disease 62, 194
Chemoprophylaxis, malarial 25
Chickenpox 143
Child abuse 183
Chloride-losing diarrhoea 90
Cholera 171
Chronic granulomatous disease 62, 159, 160, 194
Chronic mucocutaneous candidiasis 62, 106
Circulation 9
Cirrhosis 108
Coarctation of the aorta 75, 76, 77, 201
Cockayne syndrome 154, 160
Coeliac disease 91, 92, 93, 200
Coloboma 29, 160
Common carotid artery 1
Complement system 34, 193
Congenital myopathies 195
Congenital adrenal hyperplasia 84, 106, 108, 144, 201
Congenital adenomatoid lung malformation 55
Congenital diaphragmatic hernia 199
Congenital dislocation of the hip 136
Congenital nephrotic syndrome 84
Congenital talipes equinovarus 136
Congestive heart failure 93
Conn's syndrome 84
Contraindications to immunisation 171
Contraindications to organ donation 188
Cor pulmonale 55, 56, 57, 197
Cornelia de Lange syndrome 119, 160
Coronary artery fistula 203
Cortical blindness 159, 199
Corticosteroid 62, 171
Corticotrophin releasing factor-releasing neurones 6
CPAP 9, 45
Cranial nerves 1
Cranial nerve nuclei 116
Cranio-synostosis 117
Craniopharyngioma 70, 107, 108, 204

Crohn's disease 90, 92, 93, 155
Cruzon syndrome 130, 197
Cushing's syndrome 84, 105, 204
Cyanosis 77
Cyclophosphamide 23
Cystic fibrosis 54, 56, 57, 62, 92, 159, 196, 197, 204
Cystinuria 202
Cytomegalovirus 63, 146, 154

Dandy-Walker syndrome 116
Deafness 115, 126, 127, 136, 154, 160
Deficiency, alpha-1-antitrypsin 55, 92
Deficiency, factor V 198
Deficiency, factor XII 198
Deficiency, ornithine transcarbamylase 100
Deficiency, IgA 34
Deficiency, pyridoxine 23
Deficiency, vitamin A 57
Deficiency, vitamin C 198
Deficiency, vitamin K 198
Dermatitis herpetiformis 91
Dermoid cysts 42, 197
Di George syndrome 33, 62, 161, 200, 204
Diabetes 48, 204
Diabetes insipidus, nephrogenic 193
Diabetes mellitus 83, 153, 194
Diabetic mothers 46, 48
Diamond-Blackfan 62
Diaphragmatic hernia, congenital 199
Diarrhoea, chloride-losing 90
Dietary requirements 37
Diphtheria 54, 57, 143, 171
Disordered fetal swallowing 48
Disseminated intravascular coagulation 198
Distal renal tubular acidosis 83, 200
DNA-containing viruses 145
DNA manipulative enzymes 20
Down's syndrome 106, 130, 131, 160, 203
Drowning 188
Drug abuse, maternal 45
Dubowitz score 116
Duchenne muscular dystrophy 114. 159
Duchet-Jones diagnostic categories 76
Dystrophia myotonica 114

Early neonatal death rate 166
Ebstein's anomaly 47, 75, 76, 77, 78, 188
Echolalia 127
Edward's syndrome 56, 119, 177
Ehlers-Danlos syndrome 63, 83, 194, 200

Index

Eisenmenger's syndrome 75, 77
Ellis-van Creveld syndrome 136
Encephalitis 183, 204
Encephalocoele 42, 116, 197
Encopresis 182
Endocardial fibroelastosis 76
Enuresis 182
Enzymes, DNA manipulative 20
Enzymes, liver 11
Eosinophilia 63, 155
Epiglottitis 54
Epilepsy 182
Epstein-Barr 63, 92, 145
Erb's palsy 46
Erythema nodosum 153, 155
Erythema toxicum 155
Essential amino acids 10, 19
Exomphalos 177
Extranasal mass 42
Extrinsic coagulation pathway 64
Exudates 92

Facial paralysis 41
Factor V deficiency 198
Factor XII deficiency 198
Fanconi's syndrome 62, 202, 204
Fat digestion 11
Febrile convulsions 119
Femoral nerve 1
Fetal swallowing, disordered 48
Fibrosing alveolitis, idiopathic 56
Friedreich's ataxia 194

G6PD deficiency 24
Gardner's syndrome 56
Gastric juice 10, 90
Gaucher's disease 62, 201
Geometric mean 165
Gilles de la Tourette syndrome 114
Glands, parathyroid 29
Glasgow coma scale 195, 200
Glioma 42, 108, 118, 183, 195
Glomerulonephritis 192
Glucagon 6
Glucocorticoids, adrenal 6
Glucose 6 phosphate deficiency 159
Glycogen storage disease 19, 100
Glycogenesis 100
Glycolysis 19
Glycoprotein hormones 6

Granulomatous disease, chronic 62, 159, 160
Growth charts 106
Guillain-Barré syndrome 118, 204

Haemangioma 136
Haemangioma, subglottic 57
Haemolytic uraemic syndrome 83, 194
Haemophilia A 159
Haemophilia B 159
Hartnup disease 38, 99, 154
Hashimoto thyroiditis 203
HBIG 172
Heaf test 172
Hearing 126
Heart failure, congestive 93
Heart failure in neonatal period 76
Hemihypertrophy 136
Henoch-Schonlein purpura 82, 91, 92, 192, 194
Hepatitis A 143, 154
Hepatitis, acute 108
Hepatitis B 143, 154, 171, 172, 188, 200
Hepatoblastoma 69
Hepatoblastomas 195
Hereditary angio-oedema 34
Hereditary haemorrhagic telangiectasia 194
Hernia, congenital diaphragmatic 199
Herpes simplex 63
Hib 171
High output cardiac states 78
Hirschprung's disease 93
HIV 19, 171, 172, 188, 193
Hodgkin's disease 63, 70, 93, 115, 171, 201
Homocystinuria 38, 99, 160, 202
Homoeostasis, water 7
Homozygous achondroplasia 136
Hormones, glycoprotein 6
Horner's syndrome 46
Human milk 37
Hunter's syndrome 100, 119, 159
Hurler's syndrome 62, 100, 119
Hyaline membrane disease 46, 47, 48, 199
Hyperaldosteronism 201
Hyperbilirubinaemia 48
Hypercalcaemia 57, 105
Hyperparathyroidism 92, 203
Hyperplasia, congenital adrenal 106, 108, 144
Hypertension in the neonate 201
Hyperthyroidism 105, 108, 183, 199, 201

Index

Hypertrophic cardiomyopathy 48
Hypocalcaemia 33, 48, 105, 161, 204
Hypofibrinogenaemia 198
Hypogammaglobulinaemia 56
Hypoglycaemia 48, 105, 118, 199, 201, 204
Hypokalaemia 8, 83, 108, 178
Hypokalaemic metabolic alkalosis 84
Hypomanic/manic episodes 183
Hypoparathyroidism 107, 204
Hypopigmentation 154
Hypoplastic left heart syndrome 75
Hypoplastic left ventricle 76
Hypothermia 189
Hypothyroidism 19, 105, 117, 118, 154, 203, 204

Idiopathic fibrosing alveolitis 56
IgA deficiency 34
Immune deficiency 57
Immunisation, BCG 45
Immunoglobulin 33, 205
Inactivated polio vaccine 171
Incidence 166
Incontinence 182
Infant of diabetic mother 48
Infantile polycystic disease 193
Infectious mononucleosis 63, 143
INR 198
Insulin 20
Interleukin-1 33
Internal jugular vein 2
Intrinsic coagulation pathway 64
Intubation 200
Intussusception 91
Iron 11, 62, 154, 206

Jugular vein, internal 2

Kartagener's syndrome 56, 198
Kawasaki disease 145
Kayser-Fleischer rings 91
Kernicterus 115
Klinefelter's syndrome 56, 161, 204
Klumpke's paralysis 46
Kyphoscoliosis 56, 135

Laron dwarfism 106
Laron syndrome 107
Laryngomalacia 54, 57
Lawrence-Moon-Biedl syndrome 159, 198, 199, 204
Leber's amaurosis 159, 199

Lennox-Gastaut syndrome 118
Leucoerythroblastic anaemia 69
Leukaemia 115, 171
Leukaemia, acute lymphoblastic 69
Listeria monocytogenes 143
Liver 11, 62, 206
Liver enzymes 11
Lung cyst formation 55
Lung fields, oligaemic 75
Lung malformation, congenital adenomatoid 55
Lyme disease 146
Lymphangioma 136
Lymphocytic interstitial pneumonitis 33
Lymphoma 70, 93, 115, 171, 200

Macleod syndrome 56
Macrocephaly 119
Malaria 143
Malarial chemoprophylaxis 25
Maple syrup urine disease 38, 201
Marfan's syndrome 55, 99, 130, 160, 202
Mass, extranasal 42
Maternal drug abuse 45
Maternal PKU fetal effects 160
McCune-Albright syndrome 105, 106
Mean 165
Measles 143, 145, 171, 172
Meckel's diverticulum 91
Meconium aspiration 199
Median 165
Meningitis 143
Meningococcaemia 143, 145
Metabolites, active 24
Methaemoglobinaemia 199
Methaemoglobinuria 63
Microcephaly 45, 99, 119
Midline congenital extranasal mass 42
Milk, human 37
Mitochondrial cytopathy 115
Moebius syndrome 116, 195
Mononuclear cells, atypical 63
Mononucleosis, infectious 63
Moro reflex 117
Mothers with diabetes 48
Mothers with SLE 48
Moyamoya disease 116
Mucopolysaccharidosis 19, 100
Mumps 143, 171, 172
Munchausen by proxy 183
Mycoplasma pneumoniae 144

Index

Myotonia dystrophia 159, 195

Nasal obstruction 197
Near drowning 188
Necrotizing enterocolitis 46, 47, 91
Neonatal ophthalmia 143
Neonatal thrombocytopenia 64
Neonates of mothers with SLE 48
Nephrogenic diabetes insipidus 159, 193
Nephrotic syndrome 83, 108, 198, 200
Nerve, cranial 1
Nerve, femoral 1
Neural tube defect 45
Neuroblastoma 69, 70, 105, 106, 118
Neurofibromata 136
Neurofibromatosis 105, 16, 119, 153
Neurofibromatosis I 130
Neurofibromatosis II 130
Neuroleptics 181
Neurones, corticotrophin releasing factor-releasing 6
Neutrophil count, raised 62
Nonketotic hyperglycinaemia 100
Notifiable diseases 143
Null hypothesis 165

Oculo-facial digital syndrome 160
Oesophageal opening 2
Oesophageal sphincter pressure 25
Oesophagus 1
Oligaemic lung fields 75
Ophthalmoplegia 195
Organ donation, contraindications 188
Ornithine transcarbamylase deficiency 100
Osler-Weber-Rendu syndrome 63
Osteogenesis imperfecta 135, 136
Otitis media, acute 41
Oxygen dissociation curve 8, 56

P24 antigen 193
Pancreatitis 92, 195
Paralysis, facial 41
Parathyroid glands 29
Patau syndrome 119, 177
Patent ductus arteriosus 46, 75, 76
Pauciarticular rheumatoid arthritis 134
Pendred syndrome 203
Perinatal mortality rate 166
Persistent fetal circulation syndrome 199
Persistent stridor 54
Persistent truncus arteriosus 77

Perthes' disease 135
Pertussis 206
Pharyngeal arches 29
Pharyngeal pouches 29
Phenylketonuria 99, 119, 130, 139, 159
Phenytoin 23, 118
Photosensitivity 154
Plasmids 19
Pneumothorax 55, 197, 199, 204
Polio 171
Polyarteritis nodosa 63
Polyarthritic rheumatoid arthritis 134
Polycythaemia 48
Polyhydramnios 48
Polyp 42
Population attributable risk 167
Potassium 101
Potter syndrome 193, 199
Prader-Willi syndrome 106, 160, 204
Predictive value of a negative test 167
Predictive value of a positive test 167
Prevalence 166
Primary hyperparathyroidism 200
Primary hypoparathyroidism 204
Propionic acidaemia 38
Proximal renal tubular acidosis 83
Proximal tubule 7
Pseudo-Bartter's syndrome 196
Pseudohermaphroditism 106
Pseudohypoparathyroidism 105, 107, 204
Psoriasis 153
Psoriatic arthritis 134
PTH 105
Pulmonary atresia 76, 77
Pulmonary atresia with intact septum 75
Pulmonary cystic disease 199
Pulmonary hypertension 77, 197, 202
Pulmonary stenosis 76, 77
Pyloric stenosis 178
Pyridoxine 23, 38, 202
Pyridoxine deficiency 23, 45

Rabies 172
Raised neutrophil count 62
Ramsay Hunt syndrome 41
Reactive arthritis 135
Refsum's disease 62, 118
Relative risk 167
Renal artery stenosis 84
Renal failure
Renal function of neonates 46

Index

Renal tubular acidosis 83, 196
Renin-angiotensin system 8
Respiratory distress syndrome 199
Respiratory syncytial virus 205
Restrictive lung defects 56
Retrolental fibroplasia 159, 199
Rett syndrome 117
Rheumatic fever 76
Rheumatoid arthritis 134
Rheumatoid factor 134
Ribavirin 196
Rickets, vitamin D dependent 107
Rickets, vitamin D resistant 106, 107
Rickets 117
Riley-Day syndrome 118
RNA viruses 145
Rolandic epilepsy 117
Rubella 63, 130, 143, 144, 171, 194, 199, 203
Rubinstein-Taybi syndrome 119, 130, 160

Salicylate toxicity 206
Saliva 10
Sarcoidosis 92
Schizophrenia 181
Schwachman syndrome 92
SCID 62
Scimitar syndrome 198
Scurvy 63, 194
Sensitivity of a test 166, 167
Septic arthritis 146
Septo-optic dysplasia 105, 130
Serum alpha-fetoprotein 45, 69
Serum complement 3 levels 192
Severe combined immunodeficiency syndrome (SCID) 200
Severe tricuspid atresia 76
Sickle cell disease 62, 64, 159
Silver-Russell syndrome 107
SLE 193
Sleep problems 181
Somogyi effect 204
Specificity of a test 166, 167
Speech 126
Spherocytosis 62
Spinal muscular atrophy 118
Splenic dysfunction 64
Squints 131
Standard deviation 165
Steatorrhoea 92
Stenosis, subglottic 54

Steroid therapy 172, 201
Steroids 183, 196
Stridor 57
Stridor, persistent 54
Sturge-Weber syndrome 130, 161
Subglottic haemangioma 57
Subglottic stenosis 54
Supraventricular tachycardia 188
Surfactant 9, 46
Swallowing, disordered fetal 48
Sweat tests 19
Synacthen test 107
Systemic hypertension in the newborn 201
Systemic lupus erythematosus 48, 64, 82, 92, 200, 205

T cell defect 33
T cell deficiency 161
Talipes equinovarus, congenital 136
Tardive dyskinesia 181
Tay-Sach's syndrome 119
Teratogens 47
Tetanus 171, 172
Tetralogy of Fallot 76, 77, 161
Thalassaemia 62, 159
Thanatophoric dwarfism 136
Thelarche 203
Thyroid binding globulin 108
Thyroid dysfunction 105
Thyrotoxicosis 195
Tonsillectomy 57
Torticollis 137
Total anomalous pulmonary venous drainage 76
Total anomalous pulmonary venous return 77
Toxoplasmosis 63, 144
Tracheo-oesophageal fistula 177
Tracheostomy 41
Transplantation, bone marrow 62
Transposition of the great vessels 75, 76, 77
Transudative ascitic fluid 92
Treacher Collins syndrome 130, 160
Tricuspid atresia 76, 77
Triglycerides 11
Truncus arteriosus 161
Truncus arteriosus, persistent 77
Tuberculosis 54, 93, 105, 143, 155, 171, 188, 204
Tuberous sclerosis 69, 153, 154, 159, 160
Tumours 197

Index

Turner's syndrome 45, 56, 106, 130, 160, 203
Type IIa hyperlipidaemia 57
Typhoid 171
Tyrosinaemia 38

Ulcerative colitis 78, 92, 93, 155
Upper lobe fibrosis 54
Urea cycle 20
Urethral valves 177
Urinary tract infection 84
Urticaria neonatorum 155

Varicella/zoster 172
Vascular ring 54, 57
VATER syndrome 130
Vein, internal jugular 2
Vein of Galen 78
Vein of Galen aneurysm 78
Ventricular fibrillation 189
Ventricular septal defect 75, 76, 77
Viral hepatitis 143
Viruses, DNA-containing 145
Viruses, RNA 145
Vitamin A deficiency 57, 105
Vitamin B2 37
Vitamin B6 37, 99
Vitamin B12 38, 90
Vitamin C 37

Vitamin C deficiency 198
Vitamin D 37, 200, 204
Vitamin D excess 105
Vitamin D resistant rickets 106, 107, 159
Vitamin K 37
Vitamin K deficiency 198
Von Hippel-Lindau syndrome 69
VZIG 172

Waardenburg's syndrome 154
Water homoeostasis 7
Werdnig-Hoffman disease 100
Wheeze 54, 55, 57, 197
Whooping cough 55, 143, 171
Williams' syndrome 105, 119
Wilms' tumour 71, 106, 136
Wilson-Mikitzy syndrome 47
Wilson's disease 91
Wiskott-Aldrich syndrome 34, 62, 63, 69, 194, 200
Wolff-Parkinson-White syndrome 78, 188

X-linked recessive disorders 159
Xeroderma pigmentosum 154

Yellow fever 143, 171, 172

Zellweger syndrome 130